Passion to Heal

Passion To Heal

THE ULTIMATE GUIDE
TO YOUR HEALING JOURNEY

Echo L. Bodine

PASSION TO HEAL: The Ultimate Guide to Your Healing Journey

Published by Nataraj Publishing
1561 So. Novato Blvd., Suite A
Novato, CA 94947

Cover art and design by Greg Wittrock
Typography and text design by TBH/Typecast, Inc.

The author of this book does not dispense medical advice nor prescribe the use of any technique as a form of treatment for physical or mental problems without the advice of a physician either directly or indirectly. In the event you use any of the information in this book, neither the author nor the publisher can assume any responsibility for your actions. The intent of the author is only to offer information of a general nature to help you in your quest for personal growth.

First printing, September 1993
ISBN 1-882591-16-X
Printed in the United States of America

10 9 8 7 6 5 4 3 2

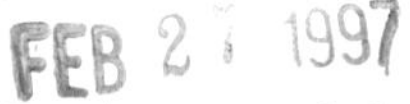

This book is printed on recycled paper containing a minimum of 50% total recycled fiber with 10% postconsumer de-inked fiber.

To the most precious healer
in my life,
Bianca Lee Bodine

Acknowledgements

I would like to thank the following people for helping me in my journey, which has led me to write this book:

My family, Ed, Mae, Scott, Nikki, Michael, Katie, Bianca, and Blake. Thank you for every lesson learned, every experience lived and every joy we've shared. We've been through a lot together, and I'm really grateful for all you've given me. I love you.

Jim Cecka. You gave me a gift of love and acceptance that I had never known before. You brought out my passion for living and loving and a playful inner child I had forgotten about. You have taught me about healing through joy and happiness. Thanks for all you've given to me. I love you.

My chiropractor and long-time friend, Dr. Marcie New. How can I ever thank you for all of the help you have given to my body, my mind, my emotions, and my soul, as I moved through this incredible journey while writing this book.

My two best friends, Melody Beattie and Ginny Miller. You've both been so wonderful and supportive while I've gone through the creation and birth of this book. I love you. Thanks for being you.

My wonderfully gifted therapist, Marilyn Meade-Moore. Thank you for taking me through my incredible healing journey.

Neil Anderson for your hours and hours of dedicated work on this book.

Hal Zina Bennett, for your great ideas and editing. Thanks for pulling it all together in order to make it happen.

The entire staff at Nataraj Publishing, for continually listening to me, encouraging me, and loving me through this whole process of getting my "baby" published.

My former partner, Wendylee Raun, for all the encouragement you've given me, your help on the book, and most of all, thanks for the great healings you've channeled to me during the many months I have worked on this book.

Bea Piper, for all the massages and help on the book.

Robb Griggs, who came into my life at the perfect time. Your positiveness and belief in me and my work is exactly what I needed.

All of my students, who pushed me and believed in me and told me this was going to happen.

My clients, who have taught me, through their own journeys, about the healing process.

Alberto Aguas, Terry Kellog, Dr. Mueller, Evelyn Baron, Virginia Miller, Tricia O'Brien, Gail Benoit, Mary Teberg, Warren Anger, Birdi, Reverend Jim Fisher and Reverend Phil Laporte, Teri Trombley, Kaye Otter, Jim Burns, Shakti Gawain, Beth Turner, Barbara Paulson Smith, Cheryl Anderson, Dick Fowler, Laura Olson, JoAnna Stamos, Grampa Boyd, Mike, Johnny, and Pam. I love you all and appreciate all that you have each given me. Thank you.

CONTENTS

SECTION II: THE SOLUTIONS

SECTION III: FROM AUTHOR TO READER

APPENDICES

How to Use This Book

Passion To Heal was written as a companion and guide for your healing journey. Section I: The Inner Work guides you through eighteen key issues that will assist you in healing those events in your life that may still be the source of pain and even physical illness. In each of these chapters I have provided some suggestions for journal work, usually in the form of simple exercises.

The first section has been written with journaling in mind, and for that reason I recommend that when you first sit down to work with *Passion to Heal* that you also have a journal in which to record your thoughts, feelings, and observations. Because I often ask you to ask your inner child to record her/his impressions, using your non-dominant hand, it is best if your journal pages are quite large. The inner child's entries usually take up a lot of space and frequently aren't neat and tidy.

Not everyone will be interested in doing the journaling work, and that's okay too. I have written all the material in this book so that any reader will find it useful, whether they do the journaling work or not.

Section II: The Solutions offers key solutions and healing methods that I have found particularly useful both in my own life and in the lives of my clients. Although this section requires no journaling, it is closely related to the material you will have covered in Section I.

Section III: From Author to Reader consists of chapters which I wanted to offer my readers in closing. It starts with a fun chapter called "Huckleberry Finn," which my inner child became very insistent about including. As the name implies, it is a reminder to keep fun in our lives, and it consists of a list of ways to get started having fun for those of us who might have forgotten how.

Next is a chapter called "Recommended Reading." If you're a person who tends to get too many things going at one time, I suggest that you sit down and read this chapter first.

In Appendix A is a list of alternative health care methods. I have tried to give you descriptions of treatments and definitions of terms that will introduce you to the world of health techniques that are now available to everyone. Knowing what is possible in this field gives you that many more healing choices. Appendix B is my personal choice of other books that I have found helpful in my own life and recommended to my clients.

If you are ill right now, I recommend that you start this book by reading the section called "If You're Sick Now," on page 169. There I offer a number of recommendations that you may find helpful even before you sit down to read *Passion to Heal* and begin the journaling work.

Remember, above all, that this is your healing journey, and the way you do this work is nobody's business but your own. Feel free to use this book and/or your journal, in whatever way you find most useful. There really are no hard and fast rules here.

Introduction: From There to Here

If attempts to find expression fail or are blocked, the repressed feelings will eventually make your body sick. It is my belief that most illnesses are caused by repressed or disowned energies within us.

—SHAKTI GAWAIN

For quite a while the Universe nudged me to write a book about the healing process. I kept pretending not to feel those nudges, remembering how much was involved with writing my first book, *Hands That Heal* (ACS Publications). Writing a book is a lot of work, and I wasn't sure how I was going to say the things that needed to be said.

As the nudges to write this book continued to get stronger I asked for what I should do to be revealed through a dream. I have learned over the years that I always get the higher guidance I need when I ask for it. For three nights in a row I dreamed I was standing in front of an Alcoholics Anonymous meeting. I was telling my story to everyone in the group.

Anyone who has ever attended an AA meeting knows that members stand up in front of the group and give testimonials about their lives, talking about how it used to be before AA and how it is now. These stories provide support for everyone who, like the speaker, is in the process of recovering.

After having this dream for the third time, I realized what I was being told—that I should share parts of my own healing journey with my readers. I should tell about growing up in an alcoholic family, being addicted to alcohol and pills, being sexually abused as a child, being an unwed mother, suffering from depression, having poor health during much of my life, and finally experiencing my own healing. This book would be about my own journey, as well as some of the many healing journeys of my clients.

With this dream in mind, I decided to begin by answering two questions that nearly every new client asks me: First, is Echo my real name? (Yes, it is.) And second, how did I get into being a healer? The second question isn't as easy to answer.

When I was seventeen years old and a junior in high school, I went to my first medium for a psychic reading. At the time, I was a typical teenager. I wanted to ask about my future husband and how many children I would have. Would I go to college? Which one?

Instead of answering any of these questions, the medium told me that I was born with psychic abilities and the gift of healing. She told me that I would be a well-known healer and psychic someday. I would teach others about their psychic abilities, would write books, and would become known throughout the world. I was stunned.

On the way home from the medium that night, I kept asking my mom: "Why me? What does all this mean? What am I supposed to do? How is it all going to happen?"

The medium knew other things, like the fact that my father was at home with a migraine headache. She told me to go home, lay my hands on his head and ask God to use my hands to heal his headache. When we got home, I told my dad everything the medium had said and asked him if I could put my hands on his head. He was as nervous and doubtful about this whole thing as my mother and I were. The only two healers I'd ever heard about were Jesus Christ and Oral Roberts. You can imagine how tough it was for a shy, seventeen-year-old girl to think of herself as having abilities like theirs!

My dad agreed to let me place my hands on his head and try to heal him. I did this, and within twenty seconds my hands started heating up like little heating pads and trembled a bit. I was scared to death! After about ten minutes, I felt my hands starting to cool off. I took my hands away and my dad announced that his headache was gone. Gone! No more pain!

We were all amazed by what happened. That night, I couldn't sleep a wink. I kept wondering, "Why me? What does this mean? Am I supposed to wear long, white robes and start acting really religious? Why did God give me this ability?" I felt an overwhelming sense of responsibility. I wondered if I was the only healer around and if all the sick people in the world were depending on me to heal them.

As I lay in bed that night I asked God if He would please help me understand everything. I had always believed in God, though I didn't know Him very well. Still, I felt confident that the help I was asking Him for would come.

A few weeks later, my psychic abilities began to develop. I began hearing voices—voices that called my name or presented me with a "one-liner" every now and then. I never knew when I was going to hear these voices. They would just come out of nowhere.

One night as I was returning from a friend's home about 1:30 in the morning, I was about to turn onto Highway 5, which was the fastest way home. I heard a voice say, "Take Highway 7." The voice seemed so real that I looked in the back seat to see who was there, but nobody was to be seen. As I approached the Highway 5 turnoff, I could not understand why I should take Highway 7, since it was a much longer way to go. I decided to take the shorter route, but as I started to make the turn I could feel something holding the steering wheel, preventing me from doing so.

I continued toward Highway 7 and then, right across from an all-night gas station, my car had a flat tire. My first reaction was that this was real *Twilight Zone* material. Had I taken Highway 5, which was one of the most sparsely traveled and poorly lit highways in the area, I might have been stranded for a couple of hours.

The voices I'd heard that night and on previous occasions continued to speak to me. I didn't know where they were coming from. But I remembered that the woman who'd told me about my gift had also talked to me about spirit guides who would help me along the way. Though I didn't know what this meant, I decided this might be the source of these voices.

For a long time I wandered around, afraid of those voices, wondering what I was supposed to do with my so-called gifts. In an effort to answer some of the questions I was having, my mom and I took psychic development classes. We even bought a Ouija board and consulted it. We read all of Ruth Montgomery's books. Her *The World Beyond* really helped me to start putting together some of the pieces of the psychic puzzle.

A spiritualist minister in town called my mother one day and told her about a class she was going to teach for people who were psychically gifted. She invited my mom and me to attend. We met every week for nearly a year. I learned a lot about clairvoyance (the gift of seeing visions or images with the third eye—the psychic eye), and clairaudience (hearing messages from the spirits). She taught us about auras (the energy around the body), reincarnation, and karma. The ideas of reincarnation and karma really bothered me. I didn't want to think about life as something I chose. It was easier to blame others or bad luck for the things that seemed to go wrong in my life. I sat on the fence about reincarnation for a long time.

Even as my abilities continued to develop, being "normal" remained very important to me. One of the issues that has always been difficult for me is the expectation that psychics and healers should be kind of weird—dress oddly, sound strange, speak in metaphysical "psychobabble," and live with a black cat in homes reeking of incense. I didn't want any of that for myself. For a long time, I made a lot of assumptions about spiritual healers, such as:

1. They never get sick because they are so in tune with their bodies.
2. They automatically have a close relationship with God. (It comes with the territory, so to speak.)
3. They have no great challenges in life because they are in some way privileged.
4. They meditate for several hours a day, eat a vegetarian diet, and follow a very rigid exercise program.
5. They are disciplined in their lives.
6. They don't seek material possessions because spirituality and materialism don't mix.
7. They are one step beyond being mere humans.

I'm not sure where I got all these ideas, but they were in my head and influencing my feelings about myself for many years. I felt like an incredible failure as a healer because I wasn't living up to these standards. I've had poor health all my life, and I've always had to work very hard at developing my closeness with God. My life was filled with challenges, one after another. I never did meditate for several hours a day, nor did I eat a vegetarian diet or follow a rigid exercise program. I had very little discipline in my life and I enjoyed material possessions. Everything about me was very human!

I felt inadequate about being a spiritual healer and worried that other healers knew something that I didn't. I asked God for help with this because I was always struggling with it. Within three days after I asked for this help, someone stopped by my office with a flyer announcing that Alberto Aguas, the internationally known healer from Brazil, was coming to Minneapolis to give a healing workshop. I felt compelled to attend.

The three-day workshop felt like a gift from God. Alberto and I became very close friends. He stayed in Minneapolis for a month, and each day we spent some time together. We talked about everything: our lives, our work, our beliefs. I saw the humanness in this world-famous teacher. It was wonderful!

I learned that Alberto wasn't perfect and never pretended to be. He did not live up to that list of imagined standards for healers any more than I did. He spoke openly of being on his own healing journey. Seeing his humanness was very healing for me. It freed me up, releasing me from the belief that my humanness was the reason that so many of my clients took such a long time to heal.

I felt a strong inner peace about myself. I let go of all my silly expectations, and as I began to accept my humanness, I also accepted my healing abilities. I started to see the truth about people's healing processes, that these were taking so long not because of my shortcomings but because each of us has processes we must go through. The journey of illness and healing is often our best teacher, showing us how to live our lives in a better way, and it is rare that we discover shortcuts on that path.

I have come a long way, both in healing myself and in accepting myself as a healer. Most of the time, I now feel peaceful about my work, my beliefs, and my journey. Most important, I now realize that I have always received whatever I needed along the way to accept my gifts and my humanness.

I have little doubt that my growing up in a dysfunctional family has made it particularly challenging for me to accept my abilities. It has taken me years to find a comfortable balance for myself. I worked with two psychotherapists who told me my voices were only my imagination. Two others were very supportive, however, helping me to accept my abilities.

One of the toughest challenges of my past twenty-four years has been learning how to live peacefully with my gifts, accepting my psychic abilities while living a normal life. Even now, whenever I fill out an application for services such as banking or other things, I flinch when I have to write in my occupation. However, I have found that the more I accept my abilities, the more the world around me accepts them as well.

In the early years, when I was still supporting myself at regular jobs, I did my psychic work in the evenings and on weekends. I was very selective about whom I told of my psychic abilities. I learned early on that many people weren't comfortable about it. Some were afraid it might be evil to be psychic. Many people assumed I could read their minds, and they were afraid because this often forced them to look at their own beliefs and feelings. For all these reasons people would squirm when I told them of my abilities, so for a long time I kept them very private. It is now twelve years since I decided to come out of the closet and do psychic work on a full-time basis.

I was not at first thrilled about this decision, and to tell the truth, it was more or less forced upon me. At the time I had been working as a barber. I had been in a car accident seven years before and had injured my back, neck, and upper arms. Cutting hair all day put a lot of stress on my back and neck muscles. Two doctors I went to advised me to find another profession. I fought the idea of changing for about nine months. I got cortisone shots in my neck and spine in order to keep going. But I kept getting messages both from the doctors and my inner voice to give up being a barber and start doing what I needed to do. Even though the voice was telling me that I would be okay financially, I wanted a sure-fire guarantee from God. I took a week off work and went to Florida to meditate and pray about the decision. I was still in a lot of pain. I had received several healings for the pain, but I knew that I had to do more than just get healings. I needed to step out with faith and give this a try. So in May 1978, I made the decision to quit barbering and do psychic work full time. Since then, the Universe has provided me with all I need, supporting my gift of healing.

Over the years, my method of working has gone through several changes, but some things have remained the same. When I do psychic readings I ask the clients to think of questions before they come in for an appointment. When they arrive, I ask them to state their questions. Then I close my eyes and through breathing and prayer, go to a calm place within myself. I always ask God to protect me and the client, and to help me bring the client accurate information that will help him or her the most.

When I first began doing psychic readings, I communicated directly with the client's spirit guides. Guides are loving, compassionate souls who want to help us. They know why we are here and what we are meant to accomplish. Through our thoughts, feelings and intuition they guide us on our life path. After I contacted these guides, they would give me information about each client.

More recently, I asked God for a spirit guide who would work with me every day, rather than communicating with different guides for every person. Shortly after my request, a guide appeared and helped me with three readings. The next day he reappeared, doing three more readings. I asked him if he was the same guide who had helped me the day before. He said that he was and introduced himself as John Joseph. He explained that he was here to make my life easier.

John was with me for five years, and we had a wonderful relationship. He was a tremendously helpful spirit, and I miss him. He was very loving, funny, and compassionate towards all people. John provided lots of important information for me and my clients, some of which I will share with you throughout the book.

Since I began working on this book, the focus of my psychic readings has shifted. Also, new guides have come to work with me. Through the information provided by these new guides, I have learned much more about the healing process and the reasons behind our health challenges. Some of the information I share with you in this book was received in this way.

This book is very different from my first one, in that the focus is not on my psychic work but on the personal journey that each of us must move through in the process of our own healing. While many books speak of the healing journey, and of the need to get down to the emotional roots of our illnesses, there were none that provided a map for this journey. And so it became my goal to provide that map, one that would be a helpful guide for anyone who was looking for a place to begin.

I would like you to think of this as a guidebook for your healing. And I highly recommend that you get yourself a book with blank pages that you can use as a journal to keep a permanent record of the exercises I suggest at the end of the chapters. Having this record of your journey can be a valuable reference for you as you do this work, one that you will turn to over and over again, reminding you of how far you have come.

Now, let's get on with our passion to heal!

SECTION I

The Inner Work

CHAPTER 1

Opening to the Healing Journey

The experience of illness is a call to a genuinely religious life. In that sense, it is for many people one of the best things that ever happened to them.
—MARIANNE WILLIAMSON

Like most people who have read the Bible, I knew about the miraculous healings performed by Jesus Christ. So when I was told at the age of seventeen that I had the gift of healing, I assumed that people would be instantly and miraculously healed when I laid my hands on them. Yet, as I look back over the past twenty-five years of doing spiritual healing, I have seen very few such instant healings. Of course, one explanation for this is that I am not Jesus Christ. But there is another reason too, one that is the focus of this book, and this is the fact that healing is a *process* that involves much more than the physical body. It is a process that must occur at many different levels —physically, mentally, emotionally, and spiritually—before we are truly healed.

Judy Pearson, one of my spiritual teachers, introduced me to the idea that most illnesses have an emotional root. She taught me that if we don't address our emotions when we feel them, and if we "stuff" them instead of expressing them, they won't just go away but will stay inside our bodies and slowly turn into physical problems. Unexpressed feelings and unresolved emotions have no other way to get our attention than for the body to become sick or be in pain.

At first this concept was difficult for me to accept. I was raised with the belief that disease and illness are just a matter of luck. If you are lucky, you don't get sick. Illness randomly strikes us and there is little or nothing we can do about it except to see a doctor when we do get ill. Worse yet is the belief, held by many, that disease is a form of punishment that comes from God. Judy Pearson was suggesting that none of these explanations were quite accurate, that we aren't just poor souls who happen to be unlucky and get sick. She was suggesting that perhaps we each have a role in creating our state of health.

In my practice as a spiritual healer and psychic, I have learned a great deal about people and their health challenges. Above all, I have seen that there are many varied reasons that we experience such challenges. For most of us, illness can be a tremendous teacher. For some, it is a way to make an exit from life here on earth.

I am continually reminded of what I have learned from Judy Pearson and writers such as Louise Hay and Alice Steadman, whose excellent books have helped me to change my thinking (see *You Can Heal Your Life,* by Louise Hay and *Who's the Matter with Me,* by Alice Steadman). Their work has helped me to see that I don't have to be a victim who is always asking why life is doing this to me, challenging my health or placing problems in my path; rather, I can start thinking in terms of what I can do to have more choices about my health.

Through my work and the changes I have experienced in my own healing journey, I am continually made aware that most illnesses do have emotional roots and until we look at the unresolved emotions in our lives, our health challenges cannot permanently disappear. We may get temporary relief from a healer, a drug, or even a surgical procedure. Our health challenge may go into remission. The physical pain may stop. But if we don't address the emotions behind the illness, they will remain in our bodies, only to rear their ugly heads at some time in the future.

That's what this book is about: the unresolved emotional pain from the time you were born until today, and what you can do about it. It's about people and their healing processes. It's about you and me. It's about no longer being victims of our health. It's about taking a really close look at the part we each play in the status of our health today.

The main focus of this book is to help you get out all the harmful things you are storing in your body so they can no longer affect your physical health or influence your life in a negative way. Whatever you are storing there is keeping you stuck in one way or another. You can go to all the doctors, healers, and health practitioners you want. You can say affirmations until you are blue in the face. You can even pray for miracles. But unless you are willing to feel the unresolved conflicts and pain, explore the negative belief systems, listen to the voices inside, and heal the hurt from your past, *you will stay stuck.* It's all in there. Your whole history is in your body, and needs to come out to be dealt with consciously.

In the pages ahead, we'll be looking at issues from this lifetime. And we'll be looking at possible solutions, such as what to do if you are sick now, whether it be having therapy, finding a good medical doctor, connecting with an appropriate support group, exploring alternatives in health care; or learning more about prayer, meditation, affirmations, forgiveness, intuition; or finding out how to make new choices in your life that will better support your healing process. We'll even be exploring how to just bring more fun into our lives.

As you read the book, and as you do the journal work that it suggests, remind yourself from time to time that this is your journey. It is an exciting one. At times it will be painful. But just remember that the pain, which you may experience as you go along, is now sitting in your body. Once you are able to release it, truly release it, you will be free of it forever!

Our illnesses can be our best teachers, guiding us not only to a new freedom from pain but to a better way to live our lives, to a fuller realization of the passion of our true gifts. Whatever you need to accept your gifts and yourself, you too can receive. Allow the process to unfold. This is perhaps the greatest purpose of the healing journey.

This book will help you on this incredible journey. Healing ourselves is not an overnight process. For most of us, our pain began long ago. When we are able to stay mindful of this and give ourselves all the time we need to do the work, we find the freedom we need to thrive as the children of God that we are.

CHAPTER 2

Illness Is a Signal for Action

Fearful as reality is, it is less fearful than evasions of reality.

—Caitlin Thomas

What would you do if a red light on the dashboard of your car suddenly went on, indicating that something was wrong? Would you wait a few days and hope that the problem would go away, in the meantime driving the car? Would you cover up the light with some black tape so that you wouldn't see the light? Or would you take the car to a person who could fix it?

When your body has something wrong with it, it has one sure way of letting you know: *pain*. Pain is the body's red warning light. What do you do when the red warning light of pain goes on in your body? Do you wait a few days and hope that the problem will go away? Do you cover it up with pain medication (like putting black tape over the red light on your car) or do you pay attention to your body's signals, going to someone who will know what's wrong?

Every ache or pain, every symptom of a physical disorder can be an early warning of trouble: constipation, diarrhea, headache, backache, numbness, bleeding, pain. Have you ever had a doctor ask you to describe the pain you're having? Do you know how many different kinds of pain the body can have? Dull, sharp, throbbing, stabbing, loud, quiet, knife-like (dull or sharp), aching, burning, biting, piercing, severe, stinging, bruising, tender, irritating, inflamed, itching.

The body has lots of little voices when something is wrong. I'm not talking about those slight aches and pains we all have now and then. I'm talking about those warning signals that last three days or longer. Why three days? I was told in a psychic reading that when the body has a minor pain that lasts at least three days, it needs to be taken seriously. This generally agrees with most medical advice, the three-day period giving your body time to heal itself, after which it may require some additional help. Something is wrong and it is trying to get your attention.

Unfortunately, most of us ignore the little signals our bodies are sending us until the problem turns into something major. The mother of a friend of mine went into the hospital on a Monday for tests because she had been having pains in her abdomen. Seven days later, she was dead. She was full of cancer. She must have been having warning signals for quite some time before she finally decided to see what was causing the problem.

So many of us don't take our bodies seriously when they are talking to us. Here are some of the excuses I have heard from clients and friends who won't take the signals from their bodies seriously:

1. I'm too busy to take the time to find out what's wrong.
2. I don't want to be inconvenienced by doctor's appointments.
3. I don't want to burden anyone, particularly the doctor.
4. I'm afraid that the doctor won't find anything wrong, and I'll be told it's all in my head.
5. I don't want to hassle with the doctor's bills.
6. I don't want to take time off from work.
7. I don't trust doctors.
8. I don't want to know what's wrong.
9. I will go *only* if my insurance company will pay the bills.
10. The pain isn't that bad.

Having had many physical problems myself, I am not a stranger to any of these excuses. But in the end, we all know none of them are really valid. John told me, "Our real partner in life is our body." When our soul comes to earth to live out this lifetime, we take on a body as a vehicle for our journey. We are given one body per lifetime.

What do you do when your body is sending you warning signals? Is the care you give your body at these times as good as the care you give your car? Have you ever noticed that when your body isn't feeling very well you can say to yourself that you don't have enough money to see a doctor, or you can't afford to take the time off from work, yet if anything goes wrong with your car you seem to be able to find the money and time to fix it? I can just hear some of you saying, "But that's different! I need my car to get around." Yes, but how far are you going to get without your body? It's the only one you've got!

There are reasons why we suffer from pain and illness. Illness is a way for us to get to know ourselves better. It's a tool to change the course of our lives. It's a teacher, a way to find freedom from the past. I strongly believe that pain and illness can be tremendous healers for us when we learn to look at them in a healthy way.

Many popular books are now available to help you identify the life changes that are associated with specific illnesses. Some that are important to me are: Louise Hay's *You Can Heal Your Life* and *Heal Your Body,* Alice Steadman's *Who's The Matter With Me* and Dennis and Marilyn Marthaler's booklet, *Illness, Thoughts, and Change.* I have found all of these to be helpful tools for finding out what might be going on behind that physical or emotional pain you're experiencing, and what changes you might make in your life as part of your healing. Although these books can be very helpful, I also encourage you to do some detective work on your own. Your body is talking to you when it hurts. It needs your attention.

The most difficult and important thing we can do when faced with a health challenge is to still our minds. We need to get away from other people, their stories, their fears, their suggestions for remedies and doctors and healers, their cures and special diets. We need to get away, to be by ourselves so that we can quiet our own fears and listen to our bodies. We need to get away so that we can listen to our own inner voice.

Whenever we are faced with a health challenge, there are solutions. Really, there are! The problem for many of us is that we know too many stories of people who had horrible experiences! It seems that as soon as we tell someone that we need surgery, that we have cancer, or whatever, they have a story *you wouldn't believe.* This causes us to get entangled in their fears as well as our own. It's very difficult to still our minds when we are full of fear.

When I am doing a healing for a client, I start by clearing from that person all the negative energy from other people that is around them. People don't intentionally send us fear-thoughts when we're sick. But they do think of us. They feel concerned, and their thoughts come to us. They intend to be loving, but we frequently get their fears and negative energy instead.

Think about the last time someone told you that he or she had cancer. When you saw that person again or talked to them on the telephone, what was your first thought? Was it, "How nice to hear from you"? Or was it, "Cancer!"? When this happens it is suddenly as if that person no longer exists. We focus on the health challenge, the illness, instead. This is disappointing for the other person as well as ourselves.

When we're faced with a health challenge, the last thing we need is to feel alone and abandoned. That's the major concern I have whenever I encounter the New Age belief that we create our own illnesses. My concern with this judgment is that it is adding feelings of guilt, shame, and loneliness to the people who are having the health challenges. Nobody needs that. What we need instead is compassion, toward ourselves or others, when facing a crisis. The person's body is talking to him or her. Something is wrong. It needs attention. It can be fixed, but we must get to the bottom of what is wrong. We can't just put a Band-Aid on it and hope that it will go away. We must listen to our bodies and respect them. They know what they need. Our job is to quiet our minds and listen to what our bodies are saying.

We choose illness on a soul level as a means of learning. There are no accidents. Webster defines accidents as "unintended events that take place." I believe that everything going on in this world of ours is in Divine Order, so I just can't buy the idea that there are unintended events taking place. Like magnets, we draw whatever accidents happen to us. Accidents are full of lessons for our souls, our minds, and our bodies.

What we need to do when first faced with a health challenge is to accept that it is truly happening. Then we need to put on our detective hats and go to work figuring out what might be going on. What is happening in our bodies? What do we need to do to heal? We need to treat ourselves and our bodies as the most important treasures we have. Remember that Jesus said, "Love your neighbor as yourself."

That means that you come first! Don't sit back and be a victim to whatever physical condition is going on. This challenge came to you for a reason. God isn't punishing you! Your health challenge is a teacher. See it as that and learn from it.

If there are negative feelings and beliefs stored in your body and you are tired of them, start right now to do what you can to free yourself from the past. The next chapter will help you identify what those possible warning signals may be.

CHAPTER 3

Negative Feelings and Beliefs

Let us be willing to release old hurts.
—MARTHA SMOCK

As a psychic and a healer, I have often seen unresolved feelings, painful memories of the past (including other lives), and negative beliefs in hundreds of clients. These are stored in our bodies until we resolve them. They are the roots of our physical problems, and their strength shouldn't be minimized. The unresolved emotional pain that we are storing inside affects our lives profoundly, threatening our health and our happiness.

It has always been difficult for me to express my feelings. When I do allow myself to experience them, I usually feel very uncomfortable. They make me nervous. I feel embarrassed when I try to express them. Some of them, such as anger or rage, even frighten me! It took quite a while in therapy before I could recognize what my feelings were—and even longer to learn how to express them. Even though I am forty-two years old, I still flinch inside when I try to tell someone what I'm feeling. A lot of this has to do with believing that my feelings aren't important and that nobody really cares about them anyway.

Many of us are afraid or embarrassed to express our feelings, so it's easier to internalize them. We stuff them. We don't let out our sadness or anger or fear or bitterness. Showing our feelings can be humiliating. Doing so can make us feel vulnerable, out of control. We're afraid that someone is going to make fun of us. They might call us a big baby or tell us that we are too sensitive, too emotional, or too dramatic.

What are your responses when someone starts talking to you about your feelings, your past, or your memories? Do you want to go smoke a pack of cigarettes or eat an entire chocolate cake? Maybe call your bookie and make a few bets or run off to the bingo parlor for a distraction? Jump on the couch with some junk food and turn the tube on? Maybe smoke a few joints or fix a few cocktails? Run out and do some shopping? I think I have had nearly every one of these responses when I have not wanted to feel my feelings.

Like many others, I have gone from one extreme to the other in dealing with my emotions. I used to give my feelings a lot of power, believing they would take control of my life if I allowed myself to experience them. I had so much anger that I was sure I would kill someone if I let it out. I had so much sadness, I thought I would cry a river if I ever let out even one tear. I also had a lot of guilt and shame. I didn't think that I could bear to look at all the reasons for these feelings. And so I tried to stay distracted for as long as possible.

When we are in emotional pain, there are many ways to dull it. As humans, most of us spend thousands of hours finding ways to hide from our pain. Distractions are everywhere. Even religion can be used as a distraction for avoiding our stored feelings and negative beliefs.

Do I mean that every feeling you ever had, or that you never expressed, is sitting inside your body? No, not every feeling. I am talking about a particular category of feelings, mainly those associated with events in your life that have created or are reinforcing *negative* beliefs you have about yourself. See the list on page 13 of some *positive* feelings. When these are felt and experienced in our lives they are a source of health.

See the list on page 13 of words often used to describe situations or negative feelings that you might experience. These reinforce negative beliefs about yourself and keep you going in circles. As you go through this list, you'll probably find that you have a strong response to some of the words while you have little or no response to others. Note in your journal which words came up for you.

You may have been brought up with certain negative belief systems about yourself, and these can also reside inside. As long as they are there, they can keep you stuck in bad jobs, abusive or unhappy relationships. They can be at the root of financial troubles or poor health. If you do nothing to change them, they will sit in your body and affect your life just like any other negative feelings. See the list on page 14 of negative beliefs that I have found in myself and my clients. As you read through the list, you might wish to note in your journal the ones that apply to you.

Positive Feelings

bliss	happiness	passion
ecstasy	joy	satisfaction
excitement	love	sympathy
fulfillment	optimism	tenderness
gladness		

Negative Feelings

abandonment	failure	pride
aggression	fear	rage
agony	being forgotten	regret
anger	fright	rejection
anxiety	frustration	remorse
arrogance	greed	resentment
bashfulness	guilt	sadness
bewilderment	hate	shame
bitterness	helplessness	sheepishness
boredom	hopelessness	sorrow
being burdened	hostility	suspicion
confusion	inadequacy	terror
depression	isolation	being trapped
deprivation	jealousy	unimportance
desperation	limitedness	unwantedness
disappointment	loneliness	unworthiness
being discounted	misery	being used
disgust	being overwhelmed	uselessness
doom	panic	being withdrawn
dread	paranoia	worry
envy	perplexity	

Negative Beliefs About Ourselves

I am:

unworthy	incompetent	incapable
unlovable	unwanted	unproductive
stupid	abandoned	undeserving
powerless	inadequate	trapped
guilty	inferior	burdensome
shameful	misunderstood	confused
bad	betrayed	weak
worthless	no good	unloved
alone	unattractive	
victimized	sinful	

Men/Women:

are inferior	have no power
create sorrow	abuse love
are undependable	abuse power
are hateful	abuse the opposite sex
like getting hurt	are victims
deserve pain	are weak

Family beliefs:

We will always be . . .

poor	misunderstood
stupid	disliked

Now let's explore how all of this works. Let's say that I believe I am incapable of making a wise decision. Possibly one of my parents or a teacher said that to me once, or repeatedly, and I have held onto it, believing it to be true. Now, let's say a situation comes up in daily life when I need to make a decision. Panic or anger about making a wrong decision are two feelings that might come up immediately for me. I might also feel foolish, ashamed, guilty, depressed, or as if I were a failure. I may feel resentful towards the person or situation forcing me to make the decision.

The problem comes when I internalize all of these feelings and beliefs. I know this is happening because I get a tight stomach or maybe a sudden headache, a spastic colon, or a pain in the back of my neck. I go through this physical, mental, and emotional torture because I have this belief that I am incapable of making a wise decision. Furthermore, I don't feel comfortable expressing my negative feelings, such as anger, humiliation, shame, guilt, or sadness. So I just keep the whole mess inside. The belief is in there along with all the feelings I have surrounding that belief. Usually, it adds up to physical trouble somewhere in my body!

Here's another example: I have a belief that I am unlovable. No one would really love me for who I am. I do everything that I can to look lovable. I spend lots of money on my outside appearance. Every time I see someone I am interested in, I get anxious or even panicky. I pretend not be interested in him because I don't want him or anyone else to know how anxious I really am. He gets the message that I'm not interested in him, and so he doesn't ask me out. He leaves me alone. This reinforces my feelings of inadequacy, fear, and panic, as well as my belief that I am unlovable. I continue to feel alone, unloved, and misunderstood.

Feelings trigger the beliefs, and the beliefs trigger the negative feelings. Back and forth they go, like a Ping-Pong ball! Those beliefs sit inside, controlling our lives, affecting our worlds outside as well as within. As in the example above, they can dictate our actions in the external world so that things which happen there seem to prove that what we're feeling is true.

If we are unable to express our feelings, they fester inside. Woody Allen once said, "I don't get angry, I grow tumors instead."

Most people, I've found, intuitively understand this process. In a recent article published in the *Minneapolis Star Tribune,* a reporter interviewed grade-school children. He asked them how they handled stress. One eleven-year-old boy said, "I don't handle my worries. I just let them hurt me inside."

How insightful and sad! The majority of us find it easier to store negative feelings inside than to go through the painful process of freeing ourselves of them. This is why I said in the previous chapter that illness is a way to get to know ourselves. It is a tool to change the course of our lives, a way to find freedom from the past. Pain, illness, and disease are our bodies' way of saying, "Help me to get unstuck. Help me to be free."

Releasing Negative Feelings

Sometimes, when we don't know what to do with our feelings, they can seem overwhelming. I would like to give you some suggestions here about what to do with your feelings rather than keeping them inside, where they can hurt you and others. The following nine suggestions are ones that I find most helpful for myself and my clients:

1. If you find that you are really angry with another person or an institution, or you have feelings of hatred, resentment, sadness, etc., write a letter. *You do not need to mail it!* The important thing is that you express exactly how you feel about that person or institution.
2. Share what you are feeling with a counselor or trusted friend. Sometimes we want someone to hear our feelings though this is not always the person with whom we have a grievance.
3. You can put a chair in front of you and pretend the person or institution is sitting in front of you. You might even tape a picture to the back of the chair. Say everything that you have ever wanted to say to them about what they did to you. Don't worry about their feelings. Take care of your feelings! If this is someone who has abused you in some way, visualize giving the offender back their shame, pain, and humiliation. Don't worry about being impolite or behaving in an "inappropriate" way. Your first priority right now is you and your feelings.
4. Sometimes, when I get really angry with someone or something, I get into my car and drive to a place where I am alone. I yell and scream as loud as I need to. I say everything I need to, until I feel an inner release of the emotions. It really works!
5. Get a plastic bat (available at toy stores) and beat your bed, couch, or a strong pillow with it. Use something soft so you won't hurt your hand.

6. Sing. Turn up the music and sing along with it, as loudly and as outrageously as you want! It's a great release! Play some of the oldies. Get those memories going. Sing!

7. Cry. Put on sad music, go to a sad movie, wallow in old memories, whatever you need to do. Just let those tears out!

8. Do something physical. This could be dancing, jogging, running, swimming, walking fast, playing a sport, bicycling, doing yard work, etc. Running on the treadmill with classical music turned up really loud is what I love to do when I'm feeling stressed, overwhelmed, or angry. Anything physical really helps!

9. Go outside, even if it's winter. Be out in nature. You will feel more grounded. You might work in a garden, mow the grass, rake the leaves, shovel snow, or go for a nature walk. If you can be outdoors and talk it out to the Universe—to the trees, birds, flowers, and rocks—it will really help to work that anxiety, fear, and anger out of your body.

Often, we get into hurting ourselves because of our unresolved feelings. This might include hitting, biting, or scratching yourself. It might include ramming your fist into the wall (hurting yourself more than the wall). It might include abusing yourself with your addictions—overeating, drinking, using drugs, overworking, spending too much money or money you don't have, or unnecessarily throwing yourself into situations that cause even more stress. Have you ever been exhausted but wouldn't accept it? You just kept on pushing and pushing and pushing. This is another form of punishment. When it comes to self-punishment, most of us are very resourceful. We may even sabotage a job offer or a relationship that we really want but don't feel we deserve.

Time to Stop the Pain

One of the most important points in this book is that your stored inner pain, memories, and beliefs have hurt you enough. It is time to stop that pain! If you come up against feelings in the exercises in this chapter that you don't know what to do with, for goodness sake don't continue to punish yourself! There are ways to get those feelings out besides hitting, starving, or stuffing yourself, creating an illness or acting them out in ways that will only cause more *dis-ease* in your life.

Try the seven suggestions above, under the heading "Releasing Negative Feelings." Start now to break those old, destructive and hurtful patterns of taking unresolved pain out on yourself. After you've released some of your feelings, give yourself a break. Praise yourself for doing good work, for possibly closing a chapter in your life. You might also want to record the experience, and any insights you might have had along the way, in your journal.

I would now like to introduce you to someone very important in your life whom you may have forgotten . . .

CHAPTER 4

The Child Within

You repress not only the pain from your childhood, but also your joy and inspiration.
—Cathryn L. Taylor

Each of us has a child within, a part of us which is sensitive, vulnerable, playful, sweet, innocent, giggly, squirmy, creative, lovable, curious, smiling, and filled with wonder. Even if you don't allow yourself to express this part, your inner child is still there—wanting and needing attention, recognition, acceptance, love, nurturance, and joy.

How do you experience joy? Do you allow yourself to get excited? Feel silly? Laugh? Do you ever take your shoes off and wiggle your toes in the water? Blow bubbles with bubble gum? Buy yourself balloons? Swing on a swing? Slide down a slide? Run through the sprinkler? Roast marshmallows on a stick over the fire? Go to an amusement park and allow yourself to see through your inner child's wondering eyes? When was the last time you flew kites or a balsawood airplane? Or colored a picture with crayons? It doesn't matter what age you are today. The child within is still in there. It needs to be recognized in order for you to feel whole and complete.

Many of us didn't get our needs met as children. We were never acknowledged for who we were. Rather, we were told who we were supposed to be. Some of us were told not to be playful, imaginative, creative, curious, giggly, or wondering. Others lost their innocence through abuse or neglect. When our childhood needs for love, nurturing, and acceptance aren't met, we grow up feeling as if there is something wrong with us. We feel lopsided. Empty. Full of holes, like Swiss cheese.

Developing a relationship with your inner child is very important for your healing process. In doing so, you will learn about yourself and will feel much more complete and whole. Whether you acknowledge your inner child or not, the fact remains that he or she continues to exist, influencing how you feel and what you do in your everyday life.

John Bradshaw, author of the best-selling books, *Bradshaw On: The Family* and *Healing The Shame That Binds You,* stated in *New Realities* magazine (July/August 1990): "The neglected wounded inner child is the major source of human misery," and that this is "the major cause of addictions and addictive behavior. When our inner child is wounded, we feel empty and depressed. Life has a sense of unreality about it; we are there, but we are not in it. This emptiness leads to loneliness. Because we are never who we really are, we are never truly present."

If your inner child was wounded, not getting all the love or positive recognition it deserved, there's a very good chance that this same inner child is still very needy today. This neediness will affect your relationships with nearly everyone around you. Maybe the only time you were ever recognized as a child was when you were playing a trick on someone or hurting them in a kidding way. Maybe you were noticed by getting yelled at or even punished, but at least you were noticed! As an adult, you may still be getting attention in similar ways. The problem is that people can't trust you. They're always on their guard because your inner child doesn't know how to ask for attention or affection in ways that are more mutually satisfying.

Perhaps as a child, you were never rewarded for the good things you did. Maybe you only heard how badly you behaved. You were never allowed to talk about your feelings. Twenty-five years later, your boss calls you into his or her office to tell you about a mistake you made. Your inner child is quite literally capable of throwing a temper tantrum. "Nobody appreciates me! Everyone hates me," it cries inside. You feel so full of rage that you could easily go out and smash up the car, hit someone, get drunk, quit your job, etc. The list of the different ways that the adult might act out the internal rage of the inner child is nearly endless. And we will continue to do this, reacting from the wounds of the inner child, until we can acknowledge it in the loving ways that it did not receive early in life.

You may have been sexually abused as a child and kept it all inside, not knowing how to talk about it or not having anyone you could trust to share what you were feeling. This made you feel powerless and confused. As an adult, maybe you act out these feelings by being very aggressive or promiscuous, desperately trying to feel sexually powerful. The inner child, in an effort to get back at the perpetrator for being made to feel so full of shame, now uses his or her sexuality to hurt everyone possible.

Maybe as you were growing up you felt no sense of protection from those around you. So the only way you could figure out to be safe was to put layers and layers of protection around yourself. You developed a weight problem. And now, no matter how many diets you try or how much weight you lose, that weight comes right back, and will continue to until your inner child can feel safe.

Perhaps when you were small, no one listened to you. So you learned to make your stories more interesting by lying or exaggerating. As an adult, you are still lying and exaggerating your stories in order to get people to listen to you. The problem is that eventually people will catch onto your lies and won't listen to you anyway!

Maybe when you were young, the only way you ever received any physical affection was to be sick. Your inner child, desperate for affection, found that he or she got something at least resembling care and affection by being sick. That same effort to get affection can carry over into adulthood, this time becoming the source of illnesses that can become life-threatening.

Are you wondering how to recognize your own inner child? My therapist gave me an excellent suggestion for doing this. Whenever you are in a situation that has brought up feelings such as fear, anger, rage, sadness, confusion, despair, hopelessness, or terror, ask yourself how old you feel. That's right! How old do you feel at the time you are experiencing these emotions? You may feel three, six, or twelve years old, or you may even feel as if you are an infant who can't speak and is totally dependent on others. This is very helpful in knowing if you're reacting from the child's or the adult's feelings.

In my own effort to understand more about how to feel, know, and embrace the inner child, I found Lucia Capacchione's book, *Recovery of Your Inner Child.* It has helped me learn a way to access my inner child in a wonderfully simple way. For those of you who are intellectual, this may be a difficult exercise, but I ask you to open your minds to the idea. Capacchione suggests having a dialogue with your inner child. She suggests taking yourself somewhere that children like to go and beginning the dialogue by letting the child within draw a picture, similar to the ones you may have drawn in kindergarten. After your inner child has drawn a picture, she suggests that you start dialoguing with the child by writing a question to him or her with your dominant hand. For instance, ask your inner child, "How are you today?" Let the child respond by writing with your nondominant hand. Here is an example of what my inner child wrote:

I am fine I am afraid
I am happy I am mad
I am sad I don't Know

Capacchione warns that we all have within us a critical parent who may try to sabotage this experience. Your critical or shaming parent may say things like:

"Hurry up, you're too slow"!

"Your penmanship is messy."

"That's a stupid thing to say."

"You're dumb."

"Your opinion is stupid."

"I have more important things to do than listen to you."

"I'm in a hurry, let's go."

"You're just a child, what do you know"?

Listen to your inner parent with the realization that the way it parents your inner child reveals something to you about how you were parented as a child. Without feeling that you have to act on what this inner parent is saying, simply take note of what it is saying. Go beyond this critical voice by paying attention to your inner child's own needs for affection and recognition; right now, these are more important than meeting the needs of the inner parent.

I would like to add that it is important to allow the child to come out at his or her own pace. When we meet a small child, we are gentle in our conversation with him or her. We don't push the child or force him or her to have a relationship with us. By the tone of our voice and mannerisms, we are trying to convey that he or she is cared for and safe. We need to treat our own inner child in the same way.

Tell your inner child that you recognize that she or he may not have felt protected but that now, as an adult, you will provide that protection. You will create a safe environment. The inner child needs to feel safe in order to really talk with you about his or her feelings. It is up to you, as the adult, now to give that child the safety, the protection, the reassurance, the attention, the acknowledgement that he or she (you) did not get earlier. Your inner child deserves to have all of these!

Are you wondering how you are going to do this? Think about any small children that you might know right now. If they came to you needing to feel safe, loved and acknowledged, how would you provide that for them? You are going to have to learn how to give this to yourself.

Inner Child Play

I would like to suggest that you buy some big crayons or markers that will help you and your inner child dialogue in your journal. Once I began dialoguing with my inner child, we went on for pages and pages!

If you have children of your own, don't use their tablets or crayons. Get a set for your own inner child! I took myself to a park that I went to as a child. I couldn't remember specific memories, but I felt childlike sitting in a park on a blanket. I immediately began drawing trees. The feeling I had was familiar, even though I hadn't experienced it for a long time. It was an excited feeling. My mind filled with ideas for my picture: the sun, the sky, a house. My imagination overtook the intellect. I switched crayons two or three times. It was fun. (See my picture on page 24.)

Of course, my critical parent was there saying, "Oh, this is ridiculous. I should be home cleaning the house or doing laundry." I jotted down these critical comments on a separate piece of paper (with my dominant hand to save time) and continued on with my picture.

Suddenly I became bored with my picture and wanted to do something else. I grabbed a pen with my dominant hand and wrote out a question to my inner child.

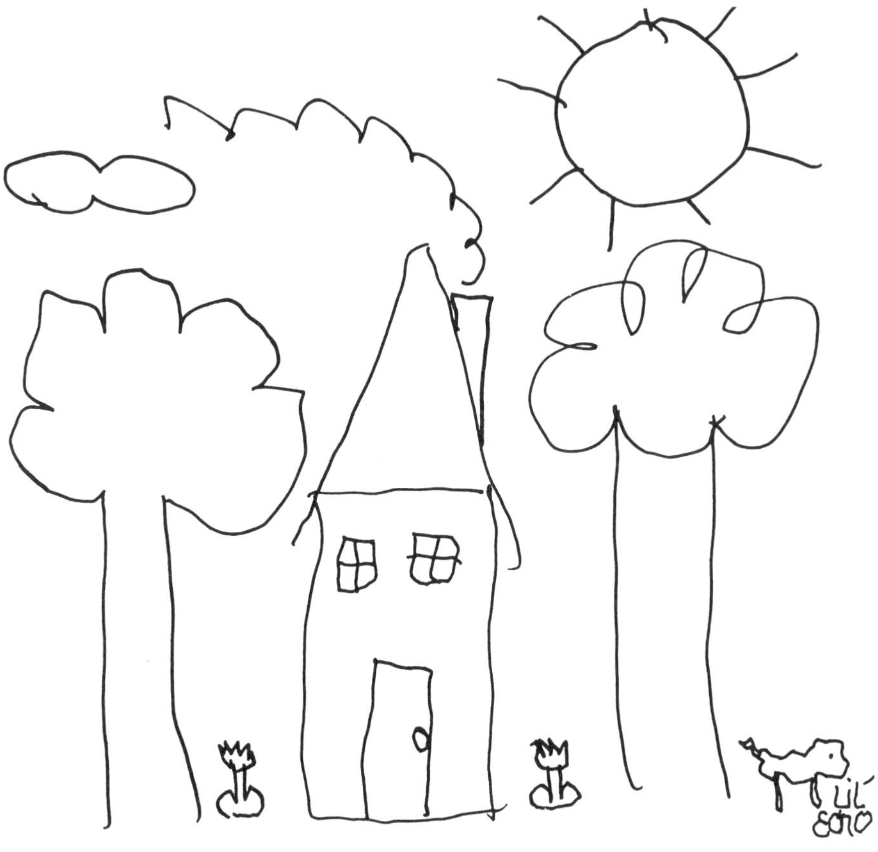

ADULT: Are you really there?

My nondominant hand grabbed a blue crayon and said, Yes!

ADULT: How are you today?

INNER CHILD: happy

ADULT: Why are you happy?

INNER CHILD: because we're at the park

ADULT: How old are you?

INNER CHILD: 4

I asked my inner child simple questions about her feelings on different subjects. Some of her replies were a single word. Others were more elaborate. Capacchione suggests asking the inner child what he or she would like to be called. Mine came up with "Little Echo," a name my dad still calls me at times today.

When you are ready to finish a dialogue with your inner child, tell him or her that you want to become more aware of her throughout your daily life. Ask her for a code, a way to let you (the adult) know that she wants or needs to talk with you. Little children love codes, remember? Mine said she would think of the color red. This has worked very well. Whenever I hear or sense an inner nudging of red, red, red, I grab my tablet and ask her, "What's up?" She always has something to say.

As you come to the end of this chapter and read the journal exercises I've included there, you may think at first that they are pretty dumb! But as silly as these exercises may seem, they are wonderfully freeing.

By doing these exercises, you will meet a very important person in your life: your own inner child from your past, the child that still exists within you. Allow yourself to feel excited about this wonderful new relationship. This child is brimming over with love for your adult self.

Love this inner child. You're the adult now. You can give your inner child everything he or she ever wanted or needed—love, recognition, acceptance, someone to listen to him or her. Acknowledging this inner child, nurturing this relationship can fill up those empty spaces inside. You will feel more complete. The unmet needs of the inner child will no longer control your life. You will feel in control of yourself and will be able to choose the way you want to live. You won't continually embarrass yourself with actions that you don't understand.

If you have not previously looked at the wounds of your inner child, he or she may not be very happy when you first make contact. Your inner child may feel very hurt, neglected, mistrustful, sad, alone, ashamed, or unwanted. Allow the child to say anything that she needs or wants to say. Give her all the time and space she needs. Your child may want to tell you how lonely she has been or how hard it was when you were little.

This inner child is not separate from you. This child is an important part of you!

JOURNAL WORK

As you start this work with your inner child, you may want to consider keeping a box of paper, crayons, and pencils set aside for your inner child work. This would be in addition to the journal you will be keeping. Let your inner child help you choose these materials, making certain there is enough so that he or she can fill up many pages with drawings or dialogue.

Think about the way small children draw and write. With your nondominant hand you will do the same, and if you only have your journal available for this you may feel somewhat reluctant to fill as many pages as you might want to do.

Exercise 1
Draw a Picture

On a separate sheet of paper, or in your journal, ask your inner child to draw a picture. Use your nondominant hand to express your inner child. Let the child pick out whatever color crayon it wants.

If your inner child is angry, she may draw an unhappy or angry picture, a mean or scary picture. Assure your inner child that this is okay. He or she can express anything they wish.

Exercise 2
Dialogue With Your Inner Child

After you are done drawing a picture, ask your child any questions that you would like. You can write this question out with your dominant hand. Then turn the pen or crayon over to your nondominant hand so that your inner child can write the answers.

You may wish to record all of these dialogues with your inner child in your journal. However, you may get quite a running dialogue going, so you might want to provide some additional scratch paper to work with rather than filling up all your journal pages with this exercise.

Exercise 3
What Is Your Inner Child's Name?

Ask your inner child what she or he would like to be called. The name your inner child comes up with may surprise you, or it may be a name you were called when you were a child.

With your nondominant hand, have your inner child record this name in your journal.

Exercise 4
A Record of Messages from Your Critical Parent

Remember to watch for your critical parent. When you hear or feel its critical messages, make a mental note of them. Then record them in your journal using your dominant hand.

Exercise 5
Your Inner Child's Secret Code

With your dominant hand, ask your inner child for a code that will let you know when he or she wants to communicate with you. Then let your inner child choose a pen, pencil, or crayon to record her or his code in your journal.

Completing a Session with Your Inner Child

As you come to the end of a session with your inner child, thank him for his picture and for sharing his feelings. Assure the child that you will continue to listen to him and that his opinion is very important to you. End your conversation in whatever way seems most comfortable to you.

As you go through this book, doing the exercises at the ends of the chapters, you'll find that many of them are written for both the child and the adult. As your adult self finishes an exercise, turn the pen or crayon over to your nondominant hand and allow the inner child to do the exercise too. The answers will sometimes be quite different from the adult's.

When the critical parent gets involved, write out its messages so that you can continue with the exercises. Recognize the critical parent as a reflection of how your inner child was treated in the past and know that you do not have to obey what it says. Just record what it says so that you will become more aware of its influence and thus become increasingly free of it.

If you decide to share the dialogue between you and your inner child with another person, make sure it is with a person who will not criticize the child in any way. This could cause the child to retreat further inside.

Having once begun dialoguing with your inner child, you will find you can use this tool throughout the day to help heal its wounds. Sometimes, of course, it won't be convenient or appropriate to grab your scribble pad or journal and ask the inner child what is wrong. However, as soon as possible, I would suggesting getting into a dialogue with your inner child about whatever situation arose, openly discussing whatever feelings you experienced. This is a wonderful way to get to know yourself and to see how you are reacting from the wounds of that child within you. As your inner child heals, so also will you heal.

CHAPTER 5

In the Beginning

A journey of a thousand miles must begin with a single step.

—Lao-tzu

Where do we begin in the healing process? At the beginning! Some therapists believe that the past is neither important nor relevant in a person's healing process. If you are a person who doesn't want to go back to your painful past, the chances are that you will be drawn to such a therapist. You may learn new "coping skills," how to "control" your emotions, and how to say no to the past. But this will keep you going around in circles, staying stuck right where you are. Every person I've ever known who has gone this route, whether they are friend or client, has remained stuck.

The healing process that I am describing in this book does not involve dredging up the past, rehashing it over and over, and then staying there. Instead, I'm talking about going back, honestly looking at your feelings, memories, and emotional pain, then talking about what you've discovered with a person who can help you let go of the pain that may be stuck in your body.

A man of about thirty-seven came to me for a healing involving his chronic back pain. His doctors couldn't find anything wrong, yet they had prescribed many different pain killers. He wanted a different solution. His back pain was causing problems in his marriage. He was irritable most of the time, and he had become very critical of his wife and everything she did. He no longer helped around the house. He had quit his job because of his constant pain and because he was always high on the medication.

When I placed my hands on his back, it felt "full." My impression was that it was swollen with emotions. I looked inside psychically and saw a man who was an alcoholic. He was yelling and hitting a young boy. Throughout his back I picked up pictures of an adult male beating or badgering this young boy and young man. I saw terror in the boy's eyes, and I saw his feelings of powerlessness and hatred for the man.

I asked my client if his father was an alcoholic, and he said yes. I asked him if his father beat him and yelled at him all the time. The answer to both questions was yes. I told him that all of his anger, his resentments, his fear, the trauma he suffered growing up in that environment were sitting in his back. I got a very strong sense that he needed a lot more help than I was giving him with the laying-on-of-hands healing.

I asked him if he had ever done any emotional work about his childhood. He said that he hadn't, replying that "what's in the past stays in the past." He truly believed, as so many of us do, that because our childhoods are out of sight, they are out of mind (and body). But as I have seen time after time, that simply is not true.

Many people think that going back to their past and dredging up all the pain isn't going to do any good. Unfortunately, these are usually the people who need to do it the most! Yes, it's hard. It's painful. I would rather have done a thousand other things than to go back and look at what it was I was trying so hard to forget. I spent years dodging the pain I stuffed inside. I distracted myself as much as possible from experiencing the feelings of the past and present. I believe that is why I have had as many health problems as I have since childhood.

This chapter is about your childhood. My childhood. Your beginning. My beginning. The child within you. The child within me. And this is where many physical problems, if you have them, probably got started . . . a long time ago. The hurt we experience, the pain, the abuse, the injustices we suffered as children, all get stored in our bodies if we do not let the feelings out at the time. Many of us were not taught to express our feelings because our parents and grandparents didn't know how to express theirs. We were taught to keep our mouths shut. "Kids are to be seen and not heard." "Don't whine." "Don't cry." "Don't talk back (because your opinion doesn't count)." "Be sweet." "Be cute." "Be the perfect child." "Always smile, even when you are disappointed." "If your feelings get hurt, swallow them." "Be a big boy." "Be a big girl."

In many cases, food or other rewards were used to soothe the feelings we were discouraged from expressing. For those of us who grew up in dysfunctional families—which is just about everyone, as it turns out—we never knew that we mattered or that we were lovable and acceptable. We didn't feel an inner safety or that we could trust our parents or care-givers to be there for us. The world appeared to be scary, unpredictable, untrustworthy, and inconsistent.

Every child needs to be loved unconditionally. When we don't get the love, attention, and affection we need while we are growing up, we may have difficulty with our relationships later in life. The reason is that our inner child continues to have deep, unfulfilled needs and insecurities, even though we have physically and mentally grown into adulthood.

I came to see that my own wounded inner child greatly affected my later life. At times, I reacted not from the place of being a full-grown adult but out of the neediness, confusion, trauma, wants, fears, of my inner child. I am going to ask my inner child, Little Echo, to share in her own words what life was like as a child in a dysfunctional family system. Through her words, hopefully your inner child will be encouraged to say what your childhood was like. (See "Little Echo's" story on pages 32–33.)

It is the curse of the child from a dysfunctional background to feel very protective of the family and its secrets. Being the firstborn in our family, I found this to be particularly true. Our family had a great sense of pride in being able to take care of each other and not need anyone else. Even as I write this chapter, the old curse of wanting to protect the family surfaces. I find it difficult to write these words. When I was in therapy, it was necessary for me to stop protecting the family pain and start paying more attention to my own feelings and my own needs for healing. As most others like me discover, we have to give up this misplaced sense of loyalty and protectiveness towards the family. This is necessary before we can really begin to heal the wounds that we carry into adulthood. As Little Echo said, she wished she could tell someone how afraid she was, but she didn't want anyone getting mad at Mom and Dad. Healing often begins at the moment when we, as adults, allow that inner child to express itself.

When I was a little kid, I did not know how to express my feelings and didn't want to be abandoned and punished. I didn't want to be a burden on anyone. I wanted my parents to want and need me, so I could feel some security about my existence. Most of the time, I felt no security whatsoever. The way I dealt with my emotions, as Little Echo said, was to get sick a lot. I was a nervous child. I had a lot of

Life was really scarey. I never felt safe. My dad was scarey because he was so big. My mom cried alot because she was afraid of my dad. They would fight when they drank. My dad would cry and tell me how hard life was. When they had parties first they would laugh and then my dad would cry and my mom would fall asleep. I would sit by her head and watch her breath so she wouldn't die. I was always afraid they would leave me. They said they loved me, but it just made me feel afraid. It was hard for me to have my sister and brothers because it seemed like so many people to take care of. My dad travelled alot. I wish he was home more, except for when he got mad or got drunk. He would get mad when we made to much noise. My mom would get nervous and get headaches. It was always scarey because I never knew what was going to happen. I was sick alot and I got to stay home alot with my mom. I liked to be with my

stomach aches, headaches, and sore throats. I suffered from constipation all the time, and I wet my bed until I was in my teens.

There was emotional, physical, and sexual abuse in our dysfunctional family system. It has been difficult for me over the years to be open, with myself or others, about how insane our family life became at times. I always minimized it. I always wanted to protect myself from being abandoned, so I wouldn't rock the boat. But all my efforts to protect what little I had only prolonged my poor health, my poor rela-

MOM when she didn't drink. I wanted To
make my parents happy so they wouldn't
drink, but I didn't know what To do.
I played house with dolls and played school.
I wet my bed and my mom would feel bad. I
Tried To stay awake but I couldn't. I was
afraid at night. I would pray to Jesus To
help me not be afraid. I would pray To
Peter Pan To Take me and my brothers and sister
to never never land, but he never did.
I just wanted to be big. Be grown up
I didn't want To be afraid anymore.
I didn't want my mom & dad To drink and
fight. And be sad. I just wanted everything
to be okay.

tionships, my low self-worth, and the negative attitudes and feelings I came to believe about myself.

If you are anything like me, you may not even know about the abuse you suffered. Some of us do such a good job of hiding the truth from others that we end up hiding it from ourselves. In order to help me discover what had happened to me, my therapist gave me a list of abusive actions. This included actions by others as well as abusive actions we might be doing to ourselves.

Pay attention to your reactions as you read over the list. Do you find yourself minimizing any of them, perhaps making excuses for those who abused you, or telling yourself that their abuse didn't really hurt you? These tendencies to downplay what occurred are the natural reactions of anyone who has suffered such treatment. But remember, abuse is abuse. Nothing on this list is good for us. Be honest with yourself as you read over this list, reminding yourself that if you are attempting to make light of anything you read here, the chances are very good that your inner child is reacting to a deep pain that he or she suffered in the past.

Physical Abuse

Slapping, spanking, shaking, scratching, squeezing, beating with board, stick, belt, kitchen utensil, yardstick, electrical cord, shovel, hose.

Throwing, pushing, shoving, slamming against walls or objects, burning, scalding, freezing, forcing of food or water, starving, having to watch others being physically abused, overworking,

Sexual Abuse

Fondling, touching, innuendoes, jokes, comments, looking, being exposed to masturbation, mutual masturbation, oral sex, anal sex, intercourse, penetration with fingers or objects, stripping and sexual punishments, pornography—either taking pictures of you or forcing you to look at such pictures. Forcing children into sexual acts with each other, forced sexual activity involving animals, watching others have sex or be abused, sexual "games," sexual torture—burning, etc.

Verbal Abuse

Excessive guilting, blaming, shaming, name calling, putting-down, comparing, teasing, making fun of, laughing at, belittling, nagging, haranguing, screaming, verbally assaulting.

Physical Neglect

Lack of food, clothes, shelter; leaving the child alone; leaving a child who is too young in charge of others; failure to provide medical care; allowing or encouraging the use of drugs, alcohol; failure to protect a child from abuse from others.

Emotional Abuse

Being put in a double bind (no matter what you choose, it's bad for you); projection and transfer of blame (being punished for the parent's own shortcomings); alterations of the child's reality (an adult telling a child that an experience they had didn't really occur—"Mama didn't beat you. You made that up."). Overprotecting, smothering, excusing, blaming others for child's problems; fostering and encouraging low self-esteem; conditional love—"Mommy won't love you anymore if you misbehave."). Double messages (one parent telling you one thing, the other telling you just the opposite.) Refusing to talk about abuse at all.

It is estimated that one out of every eight Americans is a child of an alcoholic. That means there are approximately 28 million wounded, adult children out there! And that only includes the children of alcoholic parents. What about the rest? What about the children of sex addicts? Drug addicts? Codependents? Gamblers? Overeaters? Religious fanatics? And what about the children of parents who are emotionally unstable but don't have obvious addictions? The numbers are staggering. Where does one begin the healing process? At the beginning . . . with the first step.

Characteristics of Adult Children from Dysfunctional Families

In their book *The Secrets of Dysfunctional Families,* John and Linda Friel provide the following list of characteristics that are common to people from dysfunctional families:

1. We are people who hit age 28 or 39 and suddenly find that something is wrong that we can no longer fix by ourselves. It may coincide with the normal stage crises . . . , but its intensity and accompanying pain and confusion suggests that there are Adult Child issues beneath the surface.
2. We are people who gaze at our peers on the street or at a party and say to ourselves, "I wish I could be like her or him."
3. Or we say, "If only he knew what was really going on inside of me, he'd be appalled."
4. We are people who love our spouses and care deeply for our children, but find ourselves growing distant, detached and fearful in these relationships.
5. Or we feel that everything in our lives is perfect until our sons or daughters become chemically dependent, bulimic, run away from home or attempt suicide.
6. We are the underemployed, never seeming to be able to achieve our true work potential—stuck in jobs we loathe because we're confused, afraid, or lost.

7. We are the chemically addicted, the sexually addicted, and the eating disordered.
8. We are the migraine sufferers, the exercise bulimics and the high achievers with troubled marriages.
9. We are the social "stars" who feel terribly lonely amidst our wealth of friends.
10. Some of us grew up in chaotic families and were weaned on alcoholism, incest and physical, emotional, and spiritual abuse.
11. Some of us are especially paralyzed now because the dysfunction we experienced was so subtle (covert) that we can't even begin to put a finger on what it was that happened to us.
12. Some of us were compared to a brother or sister who did well in school.
13. Others were led to believe that we could only have worth and value if we became plumbers or doctors, electricians, lawyers or psychologists.
14. Some walked on eggshells throughout childhood because the family was poor, Dad worked two jobs, Mom raised five kids pretty much by herself, and everyone was tired and on edge most of the time.
15. Many of us were emotionally neglected because no one was physically there for us; or because they were there for us with material things but were absent emotionally.
16. Some were spoiled and smothered out of misguided love; seduced to stay in the nest years after our friends had gone out into the world and begun their adult lives.
17. Many of us are afraid of people, especially authority figures.
18. Others of us frighten people, especially our loved ones and demand that our loved ones live in our isolated worlds—controlled completely by us.
19. We are people who despise religion or who despise atheism.
20. We let others use and abuse us or we use and abuse others.
21. We are people who have only anger, or only sadness, or only fear, or only smiles.

22. We try so hard that we lose; or try so little that we never live life at all.
23. We are men and women who look "picture perfect". . . .
24. We are men and women who hit skid row and feel like we finally belong somewhere.
25. We have depression or we have rage.
26. We think ourselves into emptiness or we feel ourselves into chaos.
27. We are on emotional roller-coasters or in emotional vacuums.
28. We smile while slamming the kitchen cabinets shut because we're really angry or we slam the cabinet angrily when we're really sad.
29. We abuse ourselves but take care of everyone else.
30. When we are unhappy, we are terribly afraid to acknowledge it for fear that someone will find out that we are human; or even worse, that we are even here at all.
31. We have trouble relating to our sons, our daughters or both.
32. We can make love, but we can't get emotionally close or we can't make love at all.
33. We constantly watch others to try to find out what's okay and what isn't.
34. We feel less than some and better than others but we rarely feel like we belong.
35. We get stuck in lives our hearts never chose.
36. We hang onto the past, fear the future and feel anxious in the present.
37. We work ourselves to death for unknown purposes.
38. We are never satisfied.
39. We fear God or we expect God to do it all for us.
40. We fear or hate people who are different.
41. We get into friendships that we can't get out of.
42. We get hooked on things.

43. We project our inner conflicts onto our children.
44. We are embarrassed about our bodies.
45. We don't know why we're here.
46. We suffer as much as we can.
47. We see a police car and feel like we've done something wrong.
48. We sacrifice our dignity for false security.
49. We demand love and rarely get it.
50. We wish for things instead of going out and getting what we want or need.
51. We hope for the best, expect the worst and never enjoy the moment.
52. We feel like the rest of the human race was put here to make us feel intensely uncomfortable while eating at a restaurant alone.
53. We ask, "Where's the beef?", but unlike Clara Peller in the TV commercial, we aren't getting paid to ask. And nobody answers.
54. We run away when we fall in love or we abandon ourselves for the relationship.
55. We smother those we love, we crush those we love or both.
56. Some of us will turn the tide of history by our actions, and some of us will live in obscurity.
57. We will grow up to hate our parents, or we will keep them on the pedestals that we put them on when we were little, but we will rarely let them be the error-prone humans that we all are.
58. We feel guilty about the way our brothers or sisters were treated compared to us or we feel jealous and slighted about the way they were treated compared to us.
59. We hate Dad and overprotect Mom or we hate Mom and overprotect Dad.
60. We were sexually abused by someone when we were five years old but blame ourselves, telling ourselves that we should have known better at age five.

61. Some of us had a parent who was chronically ill when we were growing up.
62. Some of us had a parent who was mentally ill when we were growing up.
63. Some of us had no parents at all when we were growing up.
64. We are survivors, who deep down inside pray that someday life will be more than just mere survival.
65. We are lovers of life whose little child is locked inside of us, waiting to be set free."

Do any of these characteristics fit for you? Read on. . . . Here's a list of roles in a dysfunctional family system from the same authors:

The Do-er

The Do-er is always *doing*, making certain the daily needs of the family are being met, making sure the children are fed, bathed, and dressed, paying the bills, ironing the clothes, doing the shopping, taking the kids to Little League or music lessons. But because the family is dysfunctional, all this consumes the do-er's time and energy, leaving him or her little or no time for anything else. So the Do-er feels tired and lonely. She may feel that others take advantage of her, and as a result may feel emotionally neglected and empty. Such a person gets a lot of satisfaction out of being so accomplished, being able to accomplish so much, and other members of the family encourage the Do-er, either directly or indirectly. Meanwhile, the Do-er's own guilt and overdeveloped sense of responsibility keeps him or her *doing, doing, doing.*

The Enabler/Helper/Lover

The Enabler nurtures other family members and provides them with a sense of belonging. Often this person is also the Do-er, but not always. The goal of the Enabler/Helper/Lover is to keep everyone together, preserving the family unit at any cost, even if it means suffering physical violence or even death. They are always trying to avoid conflict in the family, spending a lot of time and energy trying to smooth ruffled feathers. People who take on this role are often motivated by fear of abandonment and fear that other family members cannot stand on their own two feet.

The Lost Child/Loner

The Lost Child/Loner is the one who stays to herself a lot. She may stay in her room or spend time out of doors, playing in the woods by herself. This person is actually making an effort to act out a need for separateness and autonomy which most other members of the dysfunctional family feel. But while she may spend a lot of time alone, it is not a healthy aloneness because most of her time is spent trying to escape both the family and the feelings she has around it. This person usually feels a deep sense of loneliness that she carries into adulthood—or until her early feelings are resolved.

The Hero

The Hero provides the family with self-esteem. He may go off to law school and become a famous attorney, but in his heart he may secretly feel awful because his sister is in a mental hospital and his younger brother has died of alcoholism. Heroically, he carries the family banner for all the world to see, making the family proud. But all of this is accomplished at a terrible price in terms of his own well-being, since he feels burdened by the weight of his impossible task.

The Mascot

The Mascot is often a younger child. He or she provides comic relief for the family. The Mascot uses humor to give the family a sense of playfulness, silliness, fun, and a kind of distorted joy. The cost to the Mascot is that his or her true feelings of isolation and pain never get expressed. Until he gets into recovery or another program, he remains an emotional cripple.

The Scapegoat

The Scapegoat is the person who acts out all the family's dysfunction, taking the blame for the rest of them. He may be the black sheep of the family, using drugs, stealing, getting into fights, acting out sexually, etc. All of this "bad behavior" from this one person then allows the other family members to say, "If little brother would just straighten himself up, we'd be a healthy family." The cost to the Scapegoat is that he or she may spend a lifetime caught up in negative behavior and self-abuse.

Dad's Little Princess/Mom's Little Man

This child is seduced, early on, by a parent who is too afraid or dysfunctional to get his or her needs met by other adults. Adored as long as we acted out the parent's model of the ideal, loving, talented child, we are never appreciated for who we really are, nor are our own childhood needs respected. Those of us who fell into this role as children usually ended up getting physically or emotionally abused by other adults in later life because our boundaries and our needs were not respected when we were little.

The Saint/Priest/Nun/Rabbi

This child takes on the family's religious or spiritual needs and often becomes a priest, nun, rabbi, or monk. One of the conditions that may go along with this role is to live a life of denial, particularly abstinence from sex. The family may do nothing obvious to mold the person into this role, though it is implied, subtly reinforced and encouraged. This child nevertheless grows up believing that he or she will win a sense of self-worth only if they take on the spiritual/religious needs of the family.

* * *

Do you identify with any of these roles? In your journal you might want to make some notes about which ones you identify with and why. It is also worth noting here that you might identify with a combination of these roles, being a Do-er, a Hero, and a Saint, all in one. Or you might vacillate between one role and another, being a Lost Child/Loner under some circumstances, a Scapegoat at other times. In any case, take a close look at all of these characteristics and see how they fit for you.

JOURNAL WORK

Exercise 1

A Picture of Your Past

Use your journal to begin making notes about your childhood. Use your dominant hand as you write. If you are having trouble remembering your childhood, go through some family photo albums. Ask your grandparents or old family friends if they remember any stories about you as a child. Talk to friends with whom you grew up. If you have toys or other mementos from your childhood, these can also help stimulate memories of that time.

Some of the questions you might ask yourself here are: What messages did you receive as a child about expressing your feelings? Were you encouraged to speak your mind or to keep quiet? What did you do when you felt fear, anger, sadness, discouragement, or when your feelings were hurt? Whenever you did express your feelings, did anyone listen? Did they act as if they cared what you were feeling?

Look at the ways you were taught to express, or not express, positive feelings as well as the so-called negative ones. I'm talking about positive emotions such as joy, excitement, love, and happiness. Were your needs and wants respected? Did you feel people listened to you?

Note in your journal how it feels to you now as you think back and feel your childhood memories. What sticks out as the most painful memory or memories? Did your parents want a boy and you turned out to be a girl—or vice-versa? Was the fact that you turned out to be the gender you are a disappointment to them?

If you were raised by a single parent, did you in any way feel you were expected to be a surrogate spouse? Were you allowed to be a child, or did you feel you had to be mature and responsible no matter what your age? If you had brothers and sisters, were you expected to be responsible for them?

Was there physical abuse in the family? Sexual abuse? Was there a sense in your family that you didn't need any outsiders, that all you needed was each other?

Write it all out. All of it! The resentments. The sadness. The anger. Don't concern yourself with the good times since these memories are not going to cause physical problems.

You might want to go back and review the list of negative beliefs in Chapter 3 to help you with this. Write down in your journal which negative beliefs you picked about yourself when you were a child. Write down which feelings best describe your childhood. It's really important to the healing process that you be able to recognize and name these negative beliefs. For example, they might read something like this: "I am stupid. I am worthless. I am a burden. I am unwanted. I don't count. I am in the way."

Take your time with this journal entry. And please don't think you have to do the whole thing in one sitting. What you discover here is important to your health—mentally, emotionally, and physically. If you need to spread this work out over several days or even a few weeks, that's okay.

The process you will be going through in this book is not easy. There will be times when it will be emotionally painful. You will experience a lot of feelings. You will be getting to know yourself in a different way. You will be releasing some old patterns and beliefs. Many changes will take place during the journey you will be traveling in the course of reading and working with this book. Be patient. Give yourself plenty of breaks. Even as I have been writing this book, I have had to completely walk away and do something light. Yes, we want to get to the stored pain in order to free ourselves of it. But we didn't take on that pain overnight—and we won't get rid of it overnight, either!

Exercise 2

Childhood Health History

Using your dominant hand, record in your journal any health problems you had as a child, other than the usual childhood diseases. Do you still suffer from any of them? It can be helpful to ask one of your parents if they remember any specific events that occurred around the same time that you had an illness.

Illnesses such as asthma, digestive problems and mood swings can often have strong links with early events in our lives. Sometimes these can show up quite dramatically when I begin working with clients. For example, a man with asthma came to me and when I placed my hands over his lungs I saw a stored memory of his father leaving and never coming back. The word "abandonment" flashed on and off inside his lungs, like a neon sign. When I told my client what I was seeing, he replied that, in fact, when he was three years old his father left and never returned—and this was indeed the time that his asthma attacks began!

It can be helpful to divide a page in your journal into two columns. Label the first column "Childhood Illnesses" and the second one "Emotional Events." As you go through the illnesses, list any emotional events that you feel might be associated with that illness, particularly those which occurred just prior to any symptoms you might have had.

Exercise 3

Your Inner Child's Impressions of the Past

Have your inner child choose a pen, pencil, or crayon to write with, doing so with your nondominant hand. Ask your inner child to describe his/her early life. Give yourself plenty of paper for this, even if it means using some pages outside your journal.

Try to keep the adult part of yourself out of this, except to offer your inner child reassurance that you will protect him/her. Do whatever you can to give your inner child the secure feeling that it is okay to say whatever is on her or his mind. You may, as an adult, need to ask questions from time to time. Once again, remember that we're looking for stored feelings, fears, anxieties, memories, attitudes, beliefs, and emotional pain (including memories of physical or sexual abuse).

Along the way, the critical parent is likely to surface. As it does, making comments on what your inner child is expressing, note what these comments are. I recommend that you have a separate page for these comments rather than mingling them with the inner child's work.

Finishing Up

When you are done with any or all of these exercises, I strongly recommend that you do something physical to work these feelings out of your body. Or take yourself out and do something fun. If you can't think of anything, turn to Section III, page 219 called "Huckleberry Finn." It's full of suggestions for how to have fun.

If you begin feeling a lot of pain after doing any of these exercises, be conscious of the fact that the pain you have allowed to come to the surface has been stored in your body for years and years. In letting it out, you are doing a wonderful cleansing of your body and soul. You may wish to call a friend with whom you feel comfortable sharing your pain; talk with her or him about what you are experiencing. That's what you need.

If you don't have a close friend or confidant you feel comfortable with, perhaps now is the time to start looking for a therapist.

Although this book helps you sort through the pain, you may also want to consider working with a therapist. Don't think that you have to do it alone. Ask some of your friends if they know of a good therapist. If you have health insurance, call them and ask for a referral to a person who believes in "family of origin" work. You may wish to do the exercises in this book and use them as part of any therapy you might do.

Be as loving as you can to yourself. Be gentle and understanding. You're doing a great job. Keep going!

CHAPTER 6

Secrets and SECRETS

What happens to these secrets, these painful memories that we continue to hold inside? What happens to them?

—Echo Bodine

There are two kinds of secrets: those that are conscious and those that are not conscious. In this chapter we will examine both kinds and see how each affects our lives. First, let's take a look at how damaging consciously kept secrets can be.

A good friend of mine called recently. She was very upset because the youth minister at her church had just committed suicide. She asked me if I would use my psychic abilities to see his soul clairvoyantly. She wanted some help in understanding why this popular, thirty-four-year-old minister would lie beneath the exhaust pipes of his brand new truck and take his own life. She said that he was always smiling, always there for everyone. He seemed to love life and had everything going for him. These seem to be the standard remarks made about most people who commit suicide. While not everyone who has these traits commits suicide, it does seem to be the profile of people who never show they are in pain.

I was surprised that I was able to tune into this man so soon after his death. As soon as I closed my eyes, there he was in all of his pain. John explained to me that he had been sexually abused as a young boy by two men close to him. One was his father; the other was his minister. He grew up feeling very guilty and dirty. He felt like a sinner, a very bad sinner. He said that one of the major reasons this man went into the ministry was to cleanse himself of his dirtiness. He never told anyone about being sexually abused; he was too ashamed. He felt responsible for the men's actions. John said that this young man also knew secrets of many of the men with whom he worked and couldn't take one more ounce of the pain. He wanted relief. Suicide had seemed to be the only way out.

John went on to say that the problem now was that he was not happy with his choice to take his life. He had been hopeful that getting out of his body and going to heaven would rid him of his emotional pain. However, he found that once he got there, the pain was still with him. Also, he now had more guilt for having taken his own life.

This young man had gone through his entire life protecting two men he loved very much—men who had hurt him deeply. As strange as it might seem, this man is not alone in the kinds of choices he made in his life. Many people I have seen over the years consciously choose to hang on to their hidden pain. They remember the sexual, physical, or emotional abuse that has been done to them, and they know who it was that hurt them in this way. But in no way will they let the secrets out. They tell me it is too embarrassing, too humiliating. They don't want to hurt the person who hurt them. They would rather protect their victimizer than be honest and talk about their own pain.

One client of mine is conscious of having been sexually abused as a child by her mother, but she is too embarassed to go to a therapist with it or to talk to her mother about it. She goes to great lengths not to let her mother be around her children. She cringes whenever her mother touches her. Usually after some kind of encounter with her mother, she needs to come in for a healing for a migraine headache. She does not want to get any other kind of help for this because she doesn't want to open up Pandora's box, where she knows all the dysfunction of her family is hidden. She insists that she's just fine keeping the secret.

What happens to these secrets, these painful memories that we continue to hold inside? What happens to them? Do our memory banks store them safely and neatly for us, where they can do no harm to us or anyone else? Or is it possible that our bodies hold onto them for us? Are they stored somewhere in our bodies? And if so, could they possibly be the seeds of physical illness?

Do yourself a favor. Don't minimize the pain that was done to you. I believe that our secrets chip away at the physical body until we get some therapeutic help for the emotional pain and medical help for the physical pain. Our secrets, particularly those secrets that are harboring pain, are all sitting inside our bodies.

What memories have you kept as secrets? Consider giving up those secrets. Consider writing them down in your journal. There are different degrees of secrets. You may have stolen something when you were younger. You may have witnessed something hurtful done to you or someone else. You may have overheard someone telling a lie. You may have cheated someone. You may have abused a person, an animal, or had someone abuse you. Usually, when we think of secrets, we think we've cleverly tucked them away, but most of the time, they come to mind with little or no effort the moment something reminds us of them.

As I stated earlier, there are two kinds of secrets: those we keep from others (conscious) and those we keep from ourselves (subconscious). Secrets we hide from ourselves are difficult, but not impossible, to see. I believe that the body gives us many indications, often in the form of physical symptoms, that can help us get in touch with these secrets and let them out. Let me offer you an example from my own life.

When I was thirteen years old, I became aware of my fear of boys. One part of me was absolutely boy-crazy, but another part was terrified at the thought of getting close to, or of being alone with, a boy. The thought that a boy might touch me or kiss me was terrifying. I felt weird about this because my girlfriends didn't seem freaked out by the boys.

Throughout high school, I felt the conflict inside. I wanted a boyfriend, someone I could love and who would love me in return. At the same time, I didn't want any physical contact with him. When I was fifteen, I dated a guy over the phone for months, and it was great. He lived some distance away, and it was hard for us to get together, so we carried on our relationship by phone. I loved the distance. The few times we did get together, I was always very nervous about what he would do. I did not know why I was like this.

When I was in college and became sexually involved with a man I was dating, I drank a half-pint of flavored gin to drown my fears. Many times when we were sexual, or when a man would just look at me in a sexual way, I would feel terrible feelings of hate or rage inside. There were times I would visualize hurting these men—stabbing or shooting them. While I fantasized about being powerful, I enjoyed the images of being strong and overcoming those who offended me.

My fantasies always made me feel guilty. I was always worried there was something really wrong with me. I tried to figure out why I would have strong feelings of hatred, wanting to kill someone (always male). I was too embarrassed to talk to anyone professionally about it. I talked to my mom, but she didn't know what it was about. She became concerned when I was thirteen and cried one day, because I told her I didn't want to be touched or kissed by boys. I think we both just hoped it would pass. I have a vague recollection of seeing my minister for counseling, and we determined that I was shy and had an inferiority complex.

As I grew older and felt more pressure to have a boyfriend, I would just pretend that I felt normal. I seemed always to have a boyfriend, yet I wasn't happy. There were big holes inside of me. Sex always felt so dirty and shameful. Mentally, physically, and emotionally, I had a love/hate relationship with men. I liked to think of myself as a loving person, and it was hard to be honest about the amount of hatred I had inside.

I played games with men, acting like a tease. I wanted them to need me so they would never go away, yet I also wanted them to suffer for loving me! It sounds pretty sad, looking back at it now, but at that time it was a way of life for me.

For years my body gave me clues that there was something I was holding inside. From age thirteen to twenty-nine, I was in a gynecologist's office at least once every six months, and for a couple of years, at least every other month with various female problems: I rarely ovulated, and when I did I had severe menstrual cramps, monthly vaginal infections, many ovarian and uterine cysts, painful fibroid cysts in my breasts, and vaginal hemorrhaging. All this finally led up to a total hysterectomy at age twenty-nine.

When my therapist, Mary, first suggested to me that I sounded like I had been sexually abused as a child, I felt like throwing up. My insides felt rotten. I remember holding my stomach, feeling very afraid and telling her, "No way! Even if I was, I don't want to know about it." I also told her: "Let's keep my past in the past and deal with the here and now." It took me a few weeks to become willing to look for the truth.

With Mary's help, we began the long painful process of uncovering the secrets I was keeping from myself. This was neither an easy nor a quick process. My subconscious released as much as it could, a little at a time. During the first therapy session, Mary used imagery to speak to the child within me. She spoke to Little Echo, who revealed that I was sexually molested by my sixteen-year-old, male babysitter,

Tommy. I was four years old at that time. Mary told me that I needed to deal with the rage I felt towards this person and the sexual act that had been done to me. I couldn't do it. It was too embarrassing to express my anger. I cried a lot about this, but it took years for me to get the anger out.

Despite my hesitation, Mary suggested that we go back into my childhood for more memories. It had been so painful to uncover that first situation that I told her I was sure there wasn't any more sexual abuse. While I continued in therapy with her, we talked about everything but incest or sexual abuse. I had a difficult time expressing my feelings. It was easier for me to just stay in my head and relate the cold facts and stories. She told me I wasn't going to get anywhere until I became willing to be vulnerable and give up the control of my feelings. I stopped going to therapy. As far as I was concerned, I would never be able to give up enough control to be or feel vulnerable. I had a feeling that there were more sexual abuse stories inside that needed to be expressed, but I was not ready or willing to look at them.

Seven years later, after going to two other therapists, I finally became willing to look at the issues. My ex-husband and I had a real crisis in our marriage, causing me to "hit bottom" emotionally. Mentally, emotionally, and physically I was exhausted from keeping it all inside. I felt in bondage to something awful, as if a volcano of feelings and memories were about to explode.

My chiropractor used applied kinesiology to help me understand all of the physical pain that I was in (kinesiology is explained in the chapter, "Kinesiology" in Section II, Solutions, page 176). He told me my body was in crisis and was trying to decide if she wanted to live or die. My liver was full of active cancer cells; I had terrible headaches, nausea, sore throats, jaw and dental problems, aching legs, sinuses, and colon problems. I was told that my body could not handle one more ounce of stress. He said she was "bursting apart at the seams" with unresolved issues, feelings, and memories.

That night I was completely filled with fear. I knew something was happening to me that I couldn't control. I told God that I was finally willing to do whatever was necessary to get this horrible feeling inside me *out*, once and for all.

Within forty-eight hours I was enrolled in a four-and-a-half-day, intensive clinic called Lifeworks. This literally saved my life! (For more, see "Lifeworks Clinics," Section II, page 182.) One of the things

I discovered at the clinic was more sexual abuse I had experienced as a young girl. Because the therapists created such a safe environment, my body finally felt safe to release my unconscious secrets.

Between the ages of three and twelve, I was sexually molested or abused by six different men. The worst offender was a neighbor of ours. He would come to my parents' parties and get drunk, then come into my room and lie on top of me in his drunken stupor. I would pretend that I was asleep since I didn't understand what was happening. He would move up and down on me. It felt like he had something hard in his pocket. Then he would make sounds and slobber on me. When he finally was done, he would leave. In the images that I pictured, this happened several different times.

Other images of sexual abuse came to me at random. A teacher put his hand on my breasts when I was in the sixth grade. When I was twelve years old, the man who built our house cornered me in a room and rubbed something hard in his pocket against my leg. He stared at me with a glassy look and made strange sounds. A minister I knew did basically the same thing when I was even younger (six or seven years old). He would hold me close to him, acting as if he were hugging me. Then he would rub something hard into my leg. Unclear images also came that had to do with oral sex.

I slowly became aware of the terrible feelings of shame that I had felt all my life. I once told my therapist that I felt so dirty, as if there was something really wrong with me. She told me that this feeling was shame, which was almost impossible to eliminate. Fortunately, the therapists at the Lifeworks Clinic didn't agree. They explained that it wasn't my shame I was carrying. I was carrying in my body the shame of the abusers. Those abusive men felt shameful, and as an innocent child I took on their shame. My therapists explained that this is usually the case with victims, that they take on the victimizer's feelings.

Fortunately, I was in a safe place and could let out all the rage that I had internalized for so many years: the fear I had felt as a child, the confusion, and the *whys?* I beat pillows. I screamed. I cried. I yelled so much that I lost my voice. I felt so bad for the little child inside me. All that pain that she had endured—the silence, the fear, the hatred and rage! No wonder I didn't want to be touched. No wonder I found it so difficult to trust men. No wonder my body was so sick. It had been holding in so much pain, shame, fear, guilt, sadness, and mistrust!

I also looked at many other issues that weekend—relationships, my fear of intimacy and commitment, and how I had used my body as a dumping ground for all of my feelings. I also looked at my compulsive behaviors.

There was a phenomenal difference in my body after I let those secrets out! I felt 100 percent better, even though my voice was hoarse. Three days after I returned home from the clinic, I visited my kinesiologist. He was amazed at the difference in my body, saying that he had never seen such a drastic change in the condition of a person's body. The active cancer cells were gone. I no longer had headaches from all the toxins in my system. My jaw, legs, and sinuses were back to normal. All that had been hurting me for days prior to visiting the Lifeworks Clinic had stopped. That weekend I became convinced of the damage that can go on in bodies because of neglected emotions.

One of the other participants in the clinic that weekend was a fifty-two-year-old man. He had suffered from asthma all his life. His wheezing was so loud we could hear him all the way across the dining hall. By the end of the four-and-a-half day stay, he had worked on releasing his secrets and no longer wheezed. I remember clearly when he walked into the big hall on the last day, looked around the room, and hollered, "Did anybody hear me coming?" That's when it occurred to us that his wheezing had stopped for the first time in fifty-two years. He had worked hard to successfully get at his secrets. This transformation occurred in person after person. To me it was a more significant healing weekend than any I've ever seen at a healers' convention! People looked clear. Relieved. The stress they came in with was gone. Those who had felt so hopeless now basked in hope.

Opening Inward

Your stored secrets are not necessarily the roots of all your physical problems, but they *are* going to cause some kind of physical or emotional problems. Your body does not need to be a dumping ground for other people's secrets or your own. It's vital to your health to get all those secrets out of your body. Get them out by writing them out, onto the pages of your journal.

Since you cannot be aware of subconscious secrets you may be storing, simply note any recurring physical problems you have. Identifying the physical problems is not necessarily going to reveal your hidden secrets to you, so don't try to figure out what may have caused them. I was in denial for a long time before I admitted that anything could be wrong. I never stopped to look at all the areas in my body that were experiencing problems.

To begin opening up to the secrets you are holding inside, just be still for a minute and go through your body. What pains are you aware of now? For what physical problems have you been seeing a doctor? Or not seeing a doctor? Look over the last five to ten years of your life. What are the recurring physical problems? If you were in an accident that caused long-term problems, write these down as well.

If you're feeling stuck about disclosing some secrets, ask yourself why it's so scary. What do you think would happen if you did write out that secret? Would you be punished? Who would punish you? Or would someone hate you? What is the reason you're protecting yourself or the person whose secret you are holding? Don't get down on yourself if you're feeling afraid. Be gentle with yourself!

When I think about revealing secrets I have kept inside, I think that I will get into trouble or be called a "tattletale." Neither one feels very good, so it seems easier to just keep them inside. Remember my client with the recurring migraines? It may seem easier on others if we keep the secrets inside, but it certainly isn't easier on us.

Revealing secrets that you have held in for years can be terrifying. But once released, expressed in a safe setting, such as with a counselor, a trusted friend or through journal work, we no longer have it inside us. The burden of holding it in is gone or greatly reduced. The terror can no longer exist after we've made that choice to no longer keep the secret.

JOURNAL WORK

Exercise 1

Locating Conscious Secrets

Begin this exercise by putting a line down the middle of a fresh page in your journal, making two columns. Label the first column "Conscious Secrets Stored Inside;" label the second column "Physical Aches/Pains."

Sit back, take three or four deep breaths, breathe in clarity and blow out tension and fear. Ask your body and your mind to bring to your conscious mind the secrets you are keeping inside. Write down in the first column of your journal, under "Conscious Secrets Stored Inside," whatever comes to mind. As the memories of these secrets surface, note how your body feels and record these in the column labeled "Physical Aches/Pains."

Exercise 2

Other People's Secrets

Divide a new page in your journal into two columns, this time labeling the first column "Other People's Secrets;" then label the second column, as before, "Physical Aches/Pains."

Record in the first column of this page the secrets that other people have asked you to hold for them or which you feel you must keep for them. Remember, holding onto other people's secrets can be just as draining to you, causing you to have physical problems. You may be carrying around other people's shame about their secrets, or their guilt and fear. Sometimes we take on their pain, thinking they won't have to feel it any more. Again, as you're recording other people's secrets that you are keeping stored inside, notice how your body reacts as you bring each one to mind. Write these reactions down in the second column, "Physical Aches/Pains."

Take a break after completing this exercise. Go out and do something light and fun. Go outdoors. This will help you to feel more grounded, better focused, centered, and unafraid. When you feel ready to continue, come back and we'll take a look at the next exercise, "Unconscious Secrets."

Exercise 3

Secrets of the Inner Child

Put your pencil or crayon in your nondominant hand and ask your inner child what secrets he or she is holding inside. As the adult, comfort and reassure your child, as one would do with any child who is feeling afraid. Be loving and gentle. Be understanding and patient. Reassure your inner child that you will protect him or her, that no one will scold or punish her/him. Your inner child is safe. It may be necessary to repeat your reassurances several times before you begin to feel your body calming down.

Take your time. Don't be in a hurry. The child within may have been holding onto secrets for a long time, and so is very fearful of letting them go. Give your inner child as much time as she/he needs. I can't tell you how important it is to give your inner child reassurance and more reassurance.

Be sure to supply your inner child with plenty of paper for this. When she/he finally begins letting the secrets out, they are likely to fill up many pages.

Remember that when the inner child is expressing him/herself, the critical parent is likely to jump in and start criticizing what he/she is saying or simply denying that any of it is true. You may wish to record these critical parent comments as you go along.

Exercise 4

Creating a Safe Place

When you have completed the above, dialogue with your inner child and ask what she/he now needs to feel safe. Do what you can to create an emotional atmosphere of safety and love in your mind.

* * *

After completing this work, sit back, take a few deep breaths and relax. Read these words to yourself:

> I am an adult now.
>
> I can protect myself.
>
> I will not let any more pain happen to me or my inner child.

Just sit and feel the safety of these words and their promise. Know that what you have said is true.

CHAPTER 7

Addictions and Distractions

We cannot heal our addictive mind while it is entrenched in fear and conflict. It would be like trying to get out of a Chinese finger puzzle: the harder you pull, the tighter it becomes.

—LEE JAMPOLSKY

One of the ways we deal with our unresolved pain, secrets, feelings, and negative beliefs is through addictions and distractions. My own experience of growing up in an addicted family can perhaps provide some insights into how this works. On the outside, I appeared to be super-responsible—a peacemaker, a perfectionist, a caretaker, a leader, serious-minded, confident, rigid, and in control. On the inside, I felt lonely, inadequate, afraid, confused, angry, hurt, guilty, ashamed, forever unsatisfied, afraid of making mistakes, and out of control. I acted the opposite of what I felt on the inside, not wanting people to know how inadequate I believed I was. I wanted to appear confident and strong!

By the age of nineteen, alcohol seemed to have become the perfect solution to all my inner pain and the contradictions that I was living. This occurred despite my childhood oath that I would never drink. At age eighteen, I didn't think that "just one drink" could hurt. I was on a date and didn't want to appear anything less than "cool." When my date asked me what I wanted to drink, I said, "Whatever you are having." I became very drunk and blacked out. The next day I couldn't remember a thing.

Blackouts are one of the signs of alcoholism. From that day on, I never drank in moderation. I drank straight alcohol so that I could become numb and not feel all of my internal pain and conflicts. Alcohol gave me the confidence I had never known. Also, it was a great excuse for being obnoxious; it allowed me to release all of my anger and rage. I couldn't drink every day, since my body would get too sick. But I would get drunk at least twice a week. When I wasn't drinking, I was thinking about it—always preoccupied with escaping from reality and my feelings.

At the age of twenty-three, I was rear-ended in a car accident. This turned out to be the beginning of the end of my drinking career. My neck, back, and upper arms were injured in the accident. I went to an orthopedic surgeon, who prescribed Valium to relax my muscles. He also prescribed Percodan, a powerful narcotic, and a painkiller, Talwin. I was in physical therapy every other day for several months. A neurologist put me on Fiorinal, also a painkiller, for all of the headaches that I was experiencing. Despite all the physical pain I was in, this was an addict's heaven! On days when I had a bad hangover, I could take a bunch of pills and they would make my emotional pain so much easier to bear. On days when I mixed alcohol and pills, I felt even better!

It was a frightening, frantic lifestyle, however. All the unresolved pain inside me was constantly trying to surface. Instead of looking at the issues, I would just stay high. I was terrified of my emotions. I frequently thought about suicide. At the age of twenty-four, two weeks after the death of a very close friend, I hit bottom physically, mentally, emotionally, and spiritually. I could not go on living in the pain anymore. I joined Alcoholics Anonymous (AA). This was the beginning of my healing journey.

I believe that throughout my alcoholism and pill addiction, I also acted out with other addictions. I used food to ease my pain (more on that in "The Weight Game," Chapter 14). Men and relationships were also an addiction. I was forever looking outside myself for a way to feel better. Once I got to AA, and then to Al-Anon (a 12-step support group for loved ones of alcoholics) about five years later, I really needed to work the twelve steps to recovery.

Just quitting drinking and pills wasn't enough. I had a lot of work to do on myself. I went quickly from addictions to distractions, which to me is just one step removed from addictions. Distractions are anything that distract me from feeling my feelings. A nominal list of distractions might include: TV, sports, work, religion, shopping, sex, travelling, gardening, fishing, hunting, toys, having babies, gambling, committees, pets, music, sewing, crafts, hobbies, motorcycles, other people's problems, bingo, or relationships.

An addictive person has difficulty seeing what is going on. As addicts, we can minimize ("I hardly drink a thing"), rationalize ("If you had my job, you'd drink, too!"), and deny that there is any problem. At the end of this chapter are listed the questions used by Alcoholics Anonymous, Overeaters Anonymous, and Sex Addicts Anonymous. These will help you determine if you are covering up your internal pain through addiction(s). For those of you who may wonder if you have a gambling problem, substitute the word gambling for alcohol. If you are concerned that you have a drug problem, substitute the word drugs for alcohol. To help you determine if you have distractions, look at what you do when you start to feel painful feelings. Do you immediately start searching for a distraction?

Having been an addict, I know the devastating effect of chemicals. I was always sick from taking them—regardless of whether or not I was hung-over. I had headaches and digestive and colon problems. If you are a practicing addict, your body is suffering from abuse. The toxins from your pill of choice can bring disastrous results: high blood pressure, gall bladder disease, strokes, diabetes, uterine cancer, infant mortality, etc. (This list comes from *Overeaters Anonymous, A Disease of the Body,* p. 90.)

Alcoholics and drug addicts can add to that list: liver disease; pancreatic problems; blood, stomach, colon, and kidney malfunctioning; brain dysfunctions; sleep and sexual disorders; paralysis; malnutrition; night blindness; infectious diseases; skin diseases; anemia; reproductive disorders; menstrual problems; infertility; repeated miscarriages; fetal alcohol syndrome; respiratory disorders; heart problems; and psychiatric disorders. This list goes on and on.

Once you have joined a recovery program, don't think for a second that you're "home free." The real work is only beginning. But the reward, you'll later realize, will be worth it, including freedom from the physical, emotional, and internalized pain that began your addictions.

A man in his early forties came to me for healings for a chronic cough. He said he hadn't been to a doctor because he figured that he would just be given some kind of drug and that the problem would not really be addressed. He was a recovering alcoholic and said that he didn't want to risk becoming addicted to a prescription drug.

He smoked four packs of cigarettes a day and told me that he was a heavy gambler. When I looked inside him psychically, his lungs were as black as night. I saw two smokestacks filled to the brim with smoke and toxins. His heart looked very stressed and broken. I saw an image of a woman who had broken his heart, and he was still hanging onto her and the relationship, too, even though it looked as if it had been a long time since they had been together.

Next, I saw an image of his colon, which was very heavy with feelings and old residues. It was as if a lifetime of memories, pain, and resentments was stored throughout his body. The spirits told me that the man's smoking and gambling were his way of distracting himself from all his pain.

After three healing sessions, I convinced him that he had to go to a doctor because the healings seemed to be making his cough worse. I believe the healing energy was releasing the smoke and toxins in his lungs and that his increased coughing was evidence of this. Medical tests revealed that he had cancer throughout his body. He died within a year of his first visit to me. His case is a grim reminder that we really need to clear out all those unresolved feelings and negative beliefs about ourselves.

If you are in a recovery program already, I suggest that you check out some of the other questionnaires listed. It's a very common occurrence for an addict to switch addictions—to stop using alcohol and become an overeater, or to stop overeating and become a compulsive shopper.

At one lecture I attended, a therapist said that 80 percent of all recovering alcoholics were sex addicts. In many of the different twelve-step groups that I have attended, members are frequently recovering from multiple addictions. The addict is nearly always plagued by unresolved emotional pain, negative personal beliefs, and low self-esteem. These are the things that keep the addictive cycle going. Until we completely surrender the pain and begin a new way of living, we are fighting a losing battle. Addictions work in a very cunning manner. If you are in therapy, thinking that you are working on your issues, and then getting high after your sessions, you are really just going in circles!

The chemical or other addictive substance has to go! Or the sex, the gambling, or whatever your choice of escape or distraction happens to be. It must be eliminated in order for you to really get to the root of the problem.

Examine the questionnaires on pages 60-63. If you find yourself described in any of them, ask the Universe to give you the strength and courage that you need to make the necessary changes.

An Alcoholics Anonymous Intergroup office is listed in nearly every phone book throughout the United States. Call them and ask for the number of whatever "twelve-step" group you are needing. You can break this cycle of insanity and start feeling good *now*!

Are You An Alcoholic?

To answer this question, ask yourself the following questions and answer them as honestly as you can:

1. Do you lose time from work due to drinking?
2. Is drinking making your home life unhappy?
3. Do you drink because you are shy with other people?
4. Is drinking affecting your reputation?
5. Have you ever felt remorse after drinking?
6. Have you gotten into financial difficulties as a result of your drinking?
7. Do you turn to lower companions and an inferior environment when drinking?
8. Does your drinking make you careless of your family's welfare?
9. Has your ambition decreased since drinking?
10. Do you crave a drink at a definite time of day?
11. Do you want to drink the next morning?
12. Does drinking cause you to have difficulty in sleeping?
13. Has your efficiency decreased since starting drinking?
14. Is drinking jeopardizing your job or business?
15. Do you drink to escape from worries or trouble?
16. Do you drink alone?
17. Have you ever had a complete loss of memory as a result of drinking?

18. Has your physician ever treated you for drinking?

19. Do you drink to build up your self-confidence?

20. Have you ever been to a hospital or institution on account of drinking?

If you answered yes to any one of the questions, there is a definite warning that you may be an alcoholic.

If you answered yes to any two, the chances are that you are an alcoholic.

If you answered yes to three or more, you are definitely an alcoholic.

An alcoholic is anyone whose drinking disrupts business or interferes with family or social life. An alcoholic cannot stop drinking, even though he or she may want to do so.

The "20 Questions" of Sexual Addicts Anonymous

The following are some questions to ask yourself to determine if you may be sexually addicted and to evaluate your need for the S.A.A. program:

1. Do you use sex to escape from worries or troubles or to "relax"? Do you use sex to hide from other issues in your life?

2. Are you preoccupied with your sexual fantasies?

3. Do you usually feel compelled to have sex again and again within a short period of time?

4. Do you find it difficult to be friends with other men or women because of thoughts or fantasies about being sexual with them?

5. Has your sexual behavior made you feel scared or "different"—somehow alienating you from other people?

6. Have you repeatedly tried to stop what you believed was wrong in your sexual behavior? Is your sexual behavior often inconsistent with your values?

7. Are you concerned about how much time you spend in sexual fantasies?

8. Does your pursuit of sex interfere with your normal sexual relationship with your spouse or lover?
9. Have you ever made promises to yourself or to your regular sexual partner to change, limit, or control your sexual behavior, attitudes, or fantasies, and then broken these promises over and over again?
10. Do you find it almost impossible to have sex without resorting to certain kinds of fantasies or memories of "unique" scenarios?
11. Have you found yourself compelled by your desires to the point where your regular sexual partner has resisted?
12. Has your desire for sex driven you to associate with persons or to spend time in places you would not normally choose?
13. Have you ever felt you'd be better off if you didn't need to give in to your sexual obsessions or compulsions?
14. Do you frequently feel remorse, guilt, or shame after a sexual encounter? Do you frequently want to get away from this sex partner after having sex?
15. Have your family, friendships, job, or school work suffered because of your sexual obsessions or activities? Do you take time from them to engage in sex or look for sexual adventures?
16. Have you been arrested or nearly arrested because of your sexual behavior? Have your sexual activities jeopardized your life goals?
17. Do your sexual activities include the risk of contracting disease or being maimed or killed by a violent sexual partner?
18. Has compulsive masturbation become a substitute for the kind of sexual relationship you want with your spouse or lover?
19. Does a periodic inability to have sex abate or disappear only when you engage in what you would judge to be illicit sexual activity?
20. Do your sexual behavior or fantasies ever make you feel hopeless, anxious, depressed, or suicidal?

* * *

Many people have answered yes to some of these questions, and as a result sought help through the S.A.A. program.

Are You a Compulsive Overeater

1. Do you eat when you're not hungry?
2. Do you go on eating binges for no apparent reason?
3. Do you have feelings of guilt and remorse after overeating?
4. Do you give too much time and thought to food?
5. Do you look forward with pleasure and anticipation to the moments when you can eat alone?
6. Do you plan these secret binges ahead of time?
7. Do you eat sensibly in front of others and make up for it alone?
8. Is your weight affecting the way you live your life?
9. Have you tried to diet for a week (or longer), only to fall short of your goal?
10. Do you resent the advice of others who tell you to "use a little will power" to stop overeating?
11. Despite evidence to the contrary, have you continued to assert that you can diet "on your own" whenever you wish?
12. Do you crave eating at a definite time, day or night, other than mealtime?
13. Do you eat to escape from worries or trouble?
14. Has your physician ever treated you for being overweight?
15. Does your food obsession make you or others unhappy?

How did you score? If you answered yes to three or more of these questions, it is probable that you have a compulsive eating problem or are well on the way to having one.

The Courage to Heal

If you are a practicing addict of anything, my heart goes out to you. My prayer for you is that this miserable nightmare in which you are living goes away soon and that you can get on the road to recovery. You deserve the best in life, but you will never experience it until you learn to heal the inner wounds that are causing your pain.

The fact that there are so many support groups in communities throughout the United States indicates not only that help is available to you whenever you choose to reach out but also that you are not alone. Millions of people every year enter twelve-step programs in order to seek freedom from one addiction or another, whether it's alcohol, food, sex, or any of a wide range of prescription or street drugs. Perhaps one of the most important things we have to learn on any healing journey is that our addictions are little more than an effort to distract ourselves from the pain we are hiding inside. The healing begins when we finally decide it is time to look inside ourselves and confront that pain. As challenging as that task may seem, I would like to assure you that it is far easier, and less painful, than continuing to live a life of addiction.

JOURNAL WORK

Take the time to make notes in your journal about any of your findings in this chapter. At the very least, record some of the things you felt, and any memories that came to the surface, as you were going over the above lists.

If the subject of addiction did not seem to apply to you, you might want to note how it perhaps did apply to someone in your life, either from the past or the present. Note any thoughts you have about them.

While not everyone has an obvious addiction, or even a habit that causes harm or limits their lives, we all have ways of distracting ourselves from the things that are bothering us. Note any techniques you have for distracting yourself or for getting away from uncomfortable feelings. Simply make note of these without judging them.

If you feel that you are caught up in addictive behavior of any kind, or are involved with a person who is, realize that this issue is part of your healing. Start this healing with any of the support groups and twelve-step programs I mention in this chapter. Al-Anon and Codependents Anonymous are great places to begin. Contact your local chapter of the program that applies to you or call the Alcoholics Anonymous Intergroup office nearest you for any information you might want. Take a page in your journal to record names of organizations, their meeting times, where they meet, and the name and phone number of resource people whom you discover along the way.

CHAPTER 8

Why Do Nice People Get Sick?

But, you see, the definition of nice is the people who won't express themselves, who won't express rage and anger and who internalize it and then get depressed and then get sick.

—Bernie Siegel, M.D.

How many times have you heard people ask, "Why do nice people get cancer?" Or they say, "Cancer always happens to such nice people!" Best-selling author and Yale surgeon, Dr. Bernie Siegel, explains why:

> *If you go up to any head nurse on a ward and point to two women who came in with lumps in their breasts and one is a pain in the neck and driving everyone crazy and another is this wonderful, gentle, little lady who is doing everything that everybody wants, and you ask which one has cancer, the nurse is going to say the sweet, gentle one. The nice people always get cancer. But, you see, the definition of nice is the people who won't express themselves, who won't express rage and anger and who internalize it and then get depressed and then get sick.*
>
> New Age Journal, May–June 1989

No, this doesn't mean that everyone who is nice is going to get cancer. But the truth is that there does seem to be a strong link between illness and not being able to express ourselves.

A couple of years ago, a man came to me for some healings. He'd had two heart attacks and a stroke in one year. His left side was partially paralyzed. The first thing he said to me after introducing himself was that he was a Christian and that he tried to help people as much as he could. He seemed very gentle and loving. He was a professor, an intelligent man who was sincere in his beliefs about healing. While I was channeling the healing to him, John, my spirit guide, said to me, "He's been a 'Christian' to everyone else, but forgot about himself." Indeed, this was a valuable object lesson that has served me well in my personal life as well as in my healing work.

Another client comes to mind. She came for a healing on her neck because she couldn't move her head. When I placed my hands on her, I saw the image of a man sitting in her neck. She appeared to have become "fused" with this man, always anticipating his wants and needs, always focused on him. She'd forgotten about herself. He consumed her thoughts, her time, her life.

I saw another image inside, this one of the woman herself, yelling, "Hey, you forgot about me!" There was a tremendous internal conflict going on. Should she be true to herself or to him? Who was more important? If she didn't make him the center of her life, would he leave her? It seemed too risky. The images from her body were saying, "He is a total pain in the neck, get him out of here." The guidance came to me that she needed to address her codependency and break this cycle and that she could not do this on her own. Regrettably, I don't know what happened to this woman, since I only saw her once. But if she is like many other clients I have seen with similar relationships in their lives, she did seek out and receive the kind of help she needed.

Does this sound as if I am saying that we shouldn't be nice or loving or nurturing? No, that is certainly not my intent. The problem comes when we are nice to other people at our own expense. I think it's very important to be there for others in our lives. I think it's great to be a nice person. I love nice people. But there are "nice" people and then there are nice people. Nice people take responsibility for themselves, making certain their own needs are met. Then they take the extra energy they get from this and use it to be there for others. "Nice" people take all of their energy to be there for others and end up being depleted themselves, which isn't good. Usually what follows depletion is illness, which is one of the only ways they have of feeling cared for.

The greatest loss codependents suffer is their loss of self. As "nice" people we lose ourselves in everyone else. Oftentimes when my therapist asked what my feelings or thoughts were on a particular subject, my immediate reaction was confusion. She explained that this kind of confusion means that we have fused with another person and don't know what we think or feel on our own. An example would be when my boyfriend asks me what I would like to do on Saturday night. I have two choices. One, I can take care of myself and say what it is I want to do. Or, I can fuse with him, trying to figure out what it is he wants to do and then give him that answer so he'll be happy.

By fusing in this way, the other person's needs and wants become more important than our own. When we're asked what we want, we really can't say because we've learned to make choices according to what we believe other people are thinking. As codependents, we have gotten into the habit of denying our own wants and needs, sacrificing ourselves and our health in the process.

Dr. Siegel told the interviewer in the article mentioned above that there is one simple question AIDS patients can ask themselves if they wish to gauge their chances of long-term survival. That question is: "Would you do a favor for a friend even if you really didn't want to do it?" He noted that the majority of people with AIDS answer that they would. He explained further:

> *The point is that they are out there giving up their lives to do things they don't want to do to earn conditional love out of guilt, out of feeling terrible if they didn't help their friend. And then their friend doesn't help them enough and there's more conflict and more trouble and more resentment and they make themselves miserable. When you live your life and love yourself, it's okay to say no. Long-term survivors have the ability to say no.*

Codependent people have a very difficult time putting themselves first because they believe that it's being selfish or self-centered, which is a no-no. Their self-worth is so low, they don't think they have a right to put themselves first, or to have their own opinions. Moreover, if they did have their own opinions, it is very difficult for them to imagine that anyone else would care what they believed.

A few months ago on a morning talk show, the topic was codependency. The debate was whether it was a disease or not. A very overweight woman in the audience stood up and said she did not believe in codependency and argued that it couldn't make you ill or kill you, as one of the speakers had implied. While I do not believe codependency is a physical illness in and of itself, I have seen it in both my own life and the lives of my clients and am convinced that this pattern is the emotional root for many diseases which can result in death.

I have no hesitation in saying that it is essential to your health to break the destructive pattern of codependency. I have seen in many psychic readings that the attitudes and belief systems of codependency are very harmful, not only to the codependent but to the people with whom they are fused. It's a pattern that can go on lifetime after lifetime until it is stopped. There is no freedom in codependency!

Codependency is cunning because its outer mask is loving concern, selflessness, nurturing, etc. But its roots are buried in low self-esteem. We need to heal that low self-esteem, our self-destructiveness, our self-hatred and self-denial, in order to find ourselves. We need to stop fusing with others. We need to fight for ourselves and break the pattern of losing ourselves in other people. I really do believe that this caretaking, this people-pleasing, this martyrdom, this being the rescuer to everyone else but ourselves, is causing a lot of us to get sick.

Remember what Jesus said, "Love thy neighbor and you'll be a good person." No, I'm just kidding. But I am doing so in order to point out how a lot of people don't hear what He really said, which was, "Love they neighbor as thyself." The bottom line is that we each deserve and need love and caring. Someone once said that the most valuable thing we have to give is ourselves; but if there is no self to give, the gift we try to pass along to others is going to be completely empty and of no use to anyone. In a very real way, our primary responsibility is to put ourselves first.

Learning to say no is the first step toward freeing ourselves of the bonds of codependency and to getting and staying healthy. Learning to know what we want is just as important. Codependency is not to be taken lightly. Focusing on others first, fusing with others, feeling responsible for other people's lives . . . all of it! This way of life is going to make you silently resentful and envious and angry and hateful and miserable, and you already know what happens to all that negativity sitting inside of your body. Eventually it erupts into something physically wrong.

See the list on pages 69-71 of common characteristics of a codependent person, which appears in Barry K. and Janae B. Weinhold's *Breaking Free of the Co-dependency Trap*, published in 1989 by Stillpoint Publishing, Walpole, N.H., and reprinted here by permission from the publisher. Check the list to see if codependency applies to you.

If you find that you are codependent, I would like to suggest that you find a good Al-anon group or Codependents Anonymous group to attend. Adult Children of Alcoholics groups work just as well in dealing with codependency. There also are some excellent books available that I've listed for you in Appendix B.

The last suggestion I would like to make is something that helped me break my patterns of codependency. I took a class in Assertiveness Training. This training really helped me learn how to get in touch with what I wanted and needed and how to let other people know what I required. It helped me learn how to communicate and, most importantly, it taught me how to lovingly say no—something I had to learn in order to start finding myself. Give your local YMCA or YWCA a call. They may be teaching such a class or know where you could go to attend one.

Characteristics of Codependency

If you are codependent, you tend to:

- be unable to distinguish your own thoughts and feelings from those of others (you think for and feel responsible for other people)
- seek the approval and attention of others in order to feel good
- feel anxious or guilty when others "have a problem"
- do things to please others even when you don't want to
- not know what you want or need
- rely on others to define your wants or needs
- believe that others know what is best for you better than you do
- throw temper tantrums or collapse when things don't work out the way you expect them to
- focus all your energy on other people and on their happiness
- try to prove to others that you are good enough to be loved

- not believe you can take care of yourself
- believe that everyone else is trustworthy. You idealize others and are disappointed when they don't live up to you expectations
- whine or pout to get what you want
- feel unappreciated and unseen by others
- blame yourself when things go wrong
- think you are not good enough
- fear rejection by others
- live your life as if you are a victim of circumstances
- feel afraid of making mistakes
- wish others would like or love you more
- try not to make demands on others
- be afraid to express your true feelings for fear that people will reject you
- let others hurt you without trying to protect yourself
- not trust yourself and your own decisions
- find it hard to be alone with yourself
- pretend that bad things aren't happening to you, even when they are
- keep busy so you don't have to think about things
- not need anything from anyone
- experience people and life as black and white—either all good or all bad
- lie to protect and cover up for people you love
- feel very scared, hurt, and angry but try not to let it show
- find it difficult to be close to others
- find it difficult to have fun and to be spontaneous

- feel anxious most of the time and don't know why
- feel compelled to work, eat, drink, or have sex even when you don't seem to get much enjoyment from the activity
- worry that other people will leave you
- feel trapped in relationships
- feel you have to coerce, manipulate, beg, or bribe others to get what you want
- cry to get what you want
- feel controlled by the feelings of others
- be afraid of your own anger
- feel helpless and powerless to change yourself or your situation
- think someone else needs to change in order for you to feel better

JOURNAL WORK

In your journal, make any notes you wish about the issue of codependency and how it affects you. You might want to think about specific codependent relationships in your life: For example, are there some people with whom you have a codependency, while some of your other relationships do not follow this pattern? Are there people in your life whose "niceness" makes you uncomfortable? Do you ever feel guilty about these people who, after all, are only trying to be nice to you? If you feel that you are struggling with codependent relationships, make some notes about them, describing them in terms of the above list.

Simply becoming aware of any codependent patterns in your life is a big step toward healing. But remember that just as with addictions to alcohol, food, sex or other "distractions," the roots of codependency are in the pain that we carry inside ourselves. As this pain comes to the surface, note it in your journal—what these feelings are (anger, rage, feelings of abandonment, etc.), what triggers them, and any memories they may bring up from the past.

CHAPTER 9

Pregnancy, Children, and Parenting

Some parents judge themselves quite harshly . . . We all wish we were able to live our ideals . . . yet it seems so important to be compassionate toward the person we were at that time, to be understanding and forgiving.

—MICHAEL GABRIEL

The movies always seem to make getting pregnant so romantic. The parents-to-be are usually very much in love. The woman finds a cute, clever way to tell the man how much she loves the fact that they are going to have a baby. They ride off into the sunset, have the perfect baby, the perfect life, and all live happily ever after.

Unfortunately, more often than not, getting pregnant can be a very painful experience emotionally: teenage pregnancy, pregnancy through rape, pregnancy out of wedlock, unplanned pregnancy. The pregnancy can prematurely end in a miscarriage, or be terminated by abortion. There's the pain of giving birth to a stillborn child or giving birth to a child who is considered "less than perfect," which means that there is a physical deformity or a mental disorder. Then there are the parents who go through the pain of Sudden Infant Death Syndrome (SIDS). A pregnancy may end in adoption or placing the child in a foster home. At the opposite end of the spectrum there is the pain of not being able to get pregnant.

Even under the best of circumstances, most people do not think very far ahead when they get pregnant. They don't think about the step beyond babyhood into childhood, the teenage years, and finally the adult years. What if that child is not the son or daughter they always wanted? What if the child turns out to be a disappointment or an embarrassment? I would like to address each of these areas in this chapter because I have seen in my own case, and those of many of my clients, how unresolved issues around pregnancy, children, and parenting can create some real health problems physically, mentally, emotionally—or all three.

Unplanned Pregnancy

When I was nineteen years old, I found out that I was pregnant. I had not used any means of contraception for two reasons: first, the doctor had told me that because of my poor history of ovulating I wouldn't be able to get pregnant without medical help; second, I felt guilty about having sex before marriage. Using birth control was an admission that I was no longer what I was supposed to be—a virgin.

My boyfriend, my parents, and I weighed the pros and cons of what I should do about the pregnancy. Abortion didn't feel right to me, and neither did marriage. We were so young. Our relationship wasn't the healthiest. I was terrified of being a mother and a wife.

We decided that I would go to California, stay with friends of our families, have the baby, put it up for adoption, and then come back to Minnesota. We were embarrassed to tell anyone the truth so we told friends that I was transferring to college in Palo Alto. Being pregnant and not married twenty-two years ago was a pretty shameful thing. In addition, being in California on my own was difficult because I had never been away from home prior to this. I earned money by babysitting. I wore a ring from Woolworth's and told everyone my husband was in Vietnam.

As tough as it was, I loved being pregnant, having the feeling of life inside me. I talked to my baby all of the time, holding my stomach as if I were holding him. I explained to him that I loved him more than anything and didn't want to give him up, but felt as if I should. I was so afraid that he would not feel loved. I spent many hours crying about the way it was all going to turn out. Even though I knew he was going to a good family, I was always trying to think of a way to keep him for myself. If there really was a God, I couldn't understand why a woman would have to give up her baby.

My son was born on November 20, 1968. Three days later, I returned to Minnesota, forty pounds heavier than when I had left. I had gained so much weight because I ate all of the time. I didn't know how to deal with all of my feelings around the pregnancy. Everyone thought that I was coming back from school, so no one could understand why I seemed so depressed. I had terrible "postpartum blues," which lasted for weeks.

I stayed in my room, not ever wanting to come out. I never wanted to see another man as long as I lived; I never wanted to have sex again either. However, in my state of confusion I wanted at the same time to get my baby back and marry his father. I didn't know what was right anymore. I felt miserable and moped around for about three months. Finally, my father insisted that I get a job or go back to college. He also bought a health club membership for me.

I don't remember exactly how long it took me to come out of my shell, but I ended up with a job. Also, I went on a diet and worked out at the club. However, I didn't do anything about my emotional state. So many of us think that if we just have a good job and look good on the outside, any emotional problems on the inside will go away. I did everything I could to improve myself on the outside and began my search for Mr. Right. I became almost obsessed with getting married and replacing my baby.

I am telling you this story because I know that I am not the only one who has gone through this experience. The effects of this pregnancy have lasted for at least twenty-one years. Every year since my son was born, from the beginning of October (the original estimated due date) until the 20th of November (the delivery date), I would go into a state of deep depression. I would feel a very heavy sense of loss. Mentally, I would become very preoccupied, almost as if I were someplace else, but I could not make out what was happening to me. My family and close friends noticed my behavior. Every year I would tell myself that I wasn't going to go through it again and bingo, without fail, the first week in October I would slowly start to slip into a depression. I would go to therapy early in the fall to ward it off before it began, but there seemed to be no way to control it.

I told the story over and over again, but never really got into my feelings of shame, humiliation, fear, anger, resentment, and guilt. I listed the facts—first this happened, then that happened—but I didn't talk about how I felt humiliated when people asked me about my husband or wanted to plan a baby shower for me. I felt so ashamed of myself when I ducked out of town immediately after leaving the hospital. This way I didn't have to tell anyone the truth.

I had felt like a major disappointment to my parents when I told them that I was not only being sexual, but was pregnant too! I had been fearful that my brother would no longer like me or that he would think I was a slut. I felt so bad, so ashamed when the hospital put me in a room away from the other mothers to avoid upsetting them. I didn't talk much about the incredible amount of pain I felt each time I sat outside the nursery window staring at my baby, knowing I would never touch him or be with him. I never talked about the terrible sadness I felt when I could feel a child inside me—my child—which I was going to give away. No matter how many times people said that it was such an unselfish and loving thing to put my child up for adoption, it didn't relieve that deep sense of sorrow.

All of those feelings sat in my body for years. The tapes in my body played over and over again: "I am bad. I am an embarrassment to others. I am messed up. I am no good. I can't do anything right. I am a failure. I hurt other people. I am a disgrace."

I would tell my therapists that I felt so bad, that I am really a bad person. Then I would get into my head and talk about the events that took place. I would tell the stories in great detail so they would understand why I felt the way I did, but it didn't seem to relieve the beliefs or the feelings I had. I wanted to stay away from the feelings because they were too painful to experience again. I believe today that the reason I stayed stuck for so long was because I stayed in my head and talked about the facts of my pregnancy rather than the feelings associated with my pregnancy.

When I finally started to feel my feelings about my pregnancy and the loss of my child, sharing them with my therapist, I began to heal. My therapist suggested that I really grieve my loss. At first, I responded that I had cried every year over my loss. She told me that even though I had cried, I had never really let my son go and so had never really grieved my loss. I cried off and on for the next week about this. I had to give myself permission just to cry, cry, cry . . . to get the sadness out of my body.

I've prayed that someday I would meet him and that we would be able to have some kind of relationship, but that's in the future. I've had to deal with the feelings of the past to make room emotionally for the future, whether we meet or not. It has never been up to that child I gave birth to twenty-four years ago to come back into my life and heal me. It has been up to me to heal the pain.*

Healing the Pain of Pregnancy

Do you have any negative issues around a pregnancy or pregnancies, either in your past or at the present time? Perhaps pregnancy itself was very difficult and you had no one to lean on. I had a client who still held her resentments in her uterus as the result of a pregnancy she had twenty-three years before! Her husband was very angry with her for getting pregnant and would not do a thing to help her. Even when she was in labor, he chose to go fishing.

For twenty-three years this woman held onto those resentments and finally they grew into several benign tumors in her uterus. She said she never told her husband how deeply hurt she was because she didn't want to upset him.

Start thinking about what you did when you were pregnant. Did you choose to have an abortion? Have you grieved that loss? Do you have feelings of shame or anger or guilt about having had an abortion? Have you ever dealt with the anger of having that experience? How did the abortion affect you? I have friends who, after having an abortion, say to me, "I don't want to think about it. I just want to get on with my life." I can understand that, yet I get concerned about how the stored feelings are going to affect them over time.

---

* About the time this book was going to the printer, my prayers were answered. I received a phone call from an agency that helps to bring adopted children together with their biological parents. I had hired them several months before and now they were calling to say they had found my son, Kurt Christiansen. On the day I heard his voice for the first time, I announced to him that I believed I was his biological mother and he replied, "I've been waiting for this phone call all of my life. What took you so long?" He was ecstatic and so was I! Our reunion, nearly twenty-four years after his birth, has been a joyous event for both of us, one that we have been able to share fully with his adopted parents. I would love to be able to describe all of this wonderful reunion with my readers but unfortunately there isn't room for that here. I am afraid it is going to require a whole new book.

Were you single when you found out that you were pregnant? Did you go through the pregnancy alone? What happened to the child's other parent? What are your memories? What were people's attitudes towards you? What was your attitude toward yourself? Did you feel anger, sadness, shame, guilt, remorse, hatred, etc.? All of the above?

Did you go through a pregnancy that ended painfully, such as an adoption or a stillbirth?

After your child's entrance into the world, did you discover that he or she was physically or mentally impaired? We all want to give birth to perfect children. When a parent discovers that there is something physically wrong with their child, or the child dies, most often they feel very guilty. Ashamed. Remorseful. They wonder what they could have done differently. The *if-onlys* start running through their heads. They shut down their hearts because they don't want to feel their pain, disappointment, anger, hurt, or fear. How did your friends, family, and co-workers react? How did you feel about their reactions?

If some of this is too painful for you to look at, it means that the pain is still inside, unresolved. Please do your body a favor. If you experienced a pregnancy that ended painfully, such as an adoption, a stillbirth, or a less-than-perfect child, turn to the journal work at the end of this chapter and write out your feelings.

The Other Parent

The next area to look at is the choice you made to marry or not marry because of a pregnancy. Are you happy with the way your life is turning out? Did you have different plans, goals, or dreams for yourself? Do you have resentments towards the child or your spouse? Do you feel angry or remorseful? How has this affected your relationship with God? Do you feel that God did this to you?

Single Parenthood

Are you one of the millions of people who are raising your child or children single-handedly? What a tough job! How are you coping with this? How do you feel? Do you ever feel cheated? Resentful? Angry, alone, ashamed, judged, overwhelmed, afraid, or remorseful? Is it a hardship financially?

During healings with single mothers, I have seen many negative feelings towards the child's father or the child. These feelings usually reside in the pelvic area. They need to come out of there so you can get on with your life rather than to stay stuck. I have also had male clients who are raising their children alone. They have lots of anger inside of their backs, necks, and shoulders.

The Death of a Child

Are you a parent who has gone through the pain of Sudden Infant Death Syndrome? What did you do with your feelings? Did you close up your heart? What did you do with your feelings of loss? Did you feel guilty? Do you play the *what-if* and *if-only* game with yourself? You could have so much fear of ever experiencing that kind of pain again that you have closed yourself up and are stuck there. No aliveness runs through your body. Your creativity and joyfulness are on hold. You may appear to be happy on the outside, but fear of loss can keep you a prisoner inside.

For Men

If you are a man who got a woman pregnant, how do you feel about the outcome of that pregnancy? If she terminated the pregnancy or placed the child for adoption, what did that do to you? If you married her, what did that do to you and your life? Your dreams? Your goals? Did you have any moral problems with how it all turned out? Do you doubt that the child is yours? Do you feel cheated? Trapped? Do you take your feelings out on your child because you don't know what else to do with them?

The father of my child did not want me to put the baby up for adoption. He wanted to raise him by himself. He had many feelings about the pregnancy and the outcome. He went through a lot of frustration and anger with my decision and the whole situation. It's unfortunate, but most men seem to be expected to just rise above their feelings and get on with their lives. If you are a man who has been affected by pregnancy, please don't bury your feelings or hold them inside. Do the journal work at the end of this chapter, adapting them to meet your own needs wherever necessary.

The Adoption / Foster Home Dilemma

Have you had to put your children in a foster home because it was just too difficult to keep them? I had a client who had to put all three of her children in a foster home because she could not raise them by herself. There was a lot of physical abuse in the family in which she had grown up. She was starting to get physically abusive with her children, too. She knew that it was wrong, but when she felt overwhelmed she would automatically go into a rage and start abusing the children.

This woman was experiencing an incredible amount of shame and humiliation. She was seeing a therapist once a week and coming to me for healings because the unresolved feelings of shame, anger, humiliation, guilt, fear, anxiety, remorse, and sadness were causing physical problems. She never felt very well, physically. She had several cysts in her reproductive area. Her breasts had fibroid cysts. Her energy was always low, and she was depressed.

If you have feelings concerning the placement of your children in a foster home, be sure to do the journal work at the end of this chapter.

Difficulty Getting Pregnant

The next area to look at is for those of you who, for some reason or another, cannot get pregnant but want to. How incredibly painful that must be! I can't tell you how many clients I have seen for readings and healings who cannot get pregnant! Yes, the healings can heal some of the physical blocks associated with not being able to conceive. Psychic readings can help a woman or a couple understand why they are not able to become pregnant, but it doesn't help get rid of those feelings of disappointment, sadness, anger, rage, a sense of loss, and being incomplete. In this time of modern technology, when it seems that help should be available, it is such a powerless feeling not to be able to conceive. If your spouse is the one with the problems, do you feel resentment towards him? Towards her? If so, be sure to do the exercises at the end of this chapter.

Older Children

Let's move beyond pregnancy to your children as they are growing or have grown up. Is your son or daughter the child that you always wanted? Did your children turn out to be a disappointment or an embarrassment? Did they end up being a burden on you emotionally or physically? Were they a constant thorn in your side?

If you have resentments towards one or more of your children, these feelings are going to physically hurt you. You have got to get those feelings out of your body. Do you feel jealousy or hatred towards a child? Do you feel rage, frustration, disappointment, hurt, sadness, remorse, guilt, or perhaps even envy that they have been able to do things in their lives that you haven't been able to do in yours? Please give your body a chance to unload these feelings by doing the journal work.

Being Unwanted

Were you the child of an unwanted pregnancy? How do you feel about not being wanted? That sounds harsh, but life may have been pretty harsh for you. Do you feel like a burden? As if you ruined everyone's life? Do you feel responsible for the outcome of everyone else's life?

If you came into life as the result of an unwanted pregnancy, the chances are that you will have some strong feelings about it. So take the time to do the journal work which applies to you at the end of this chapter.

Healing the Pain From Inside

Whatever your particular situation was, if the outcome wasn't what you wanted or dreamed about, you can heal from the experience. To get started with this process, do the journal work which pertains to you. It's time to begin healing the past and to get on with the goodness of life. Remember, looking at all of this is for your health's sake, not for other people. Be patient with yourself, your body. If tears come, don't hold them back. If you feel angry, yell at the whole crummy, painful situation and tell it how you feel. Beat some pillows if you need to. Just remember not to hurt yourself in this releasing process. You have been hurt enough from this pain.

JOURNAL WORK

Exercise 1

Touching Your Feelings

Put your hands on your abdomen and allow yourself to feel any emotions that are stirring up. As feelings, memories, awarenesses come up, let them flow. If tears come, let them out. If you feel angry, yell out your feelings at the situation. Take time to fully experience your feelings. Then, when you feel ready, record this experience in your journal.

Exercise 2

Being Pregnant and Single

Were you single when you found out that you were pregnant? Did you go through your pregnancy alone? What happened to the child's other parent?

What are your memories? What were people's attitudes towards you? What were your feelings about yourself? Did you feel anger, sadness, shame, guilt, remorse, hatred? All of the above? Other feelings?

Write down in your journal whatever words come up for you as these feelings surface.

Exercise 3

Pregnancies That Ended Painfully

If you experienced a pregnancy that ended painfully, such as adoption, a stillbirth, or a less-than-perfect child, let yourself feel the emotions you experienced, or are experiencing, around that issue. Let yourself open up to any anger, hurt, fear, disappointment, or pain that you are still holding in your body. Let yourself remember friends', family members', and co-workers', reactions and how you felt about them.

If any of this is too painful for you to look at, it means the pain is still there inside you, unresolved. Do your body a favor, release it from these feelings by allowing yourself to re-experience them. Each time you do this exercise, feeling your feelings and then recording them in your journal, you relieve your body of some of the burden it is carrying.

Exercise 4
Broken Dreams

Did your pregnancy change your expectations about the way you thought your life would turn out? If you had different plans, goals or dreams for yourself, do you feel any resentment toward your child, spouse, or perhaps even yourself? Do you feel angry or remorseful about the way your life is turning out? If you were raised a religious person, has this affected your relationship with God? Do you ever feel that God did this to you?

Let yourself experience any feelings that come up. Let yourself recall memories of what you had planned or dreamed for your life. Record the memories and feelings that come up in your journal.

Exercise 5
Parenting Alone

Record in your journal any feelings or memories that come to mind as a result of raising your child or children single-handedly.

Exercise 6
An Infant's Death

If you had an infant die from SIDS, or from any other cause, record your feelings about that in your journal. Record, also, any physical problems you may be having that you believe might be associated with this, so that you can come alive again.

Exercise 7
For Men Only

If you were the father in an unwanted pregnancy, allow yourself to feel the feelings you had about this. Write them down in the journal.

Exercise 8
The Adoption/Foster Home Dilemma

If you have had to place your children in a foster home or put a child up for adoption, write out in your journal what feelings you have about this. Not the stories. Don't get stuck in your head, writing out your stories. Go to your heart, your gut. Get in touch with the real feelings and record them in your journal.

Exercise 9

Inability to Get Pregnant

If you have been unable to get pregnant, what are your feelings about this? Also check out your feelings toward your partner and record anything that comes to mind.

Exercise 10

When Children Grow Up

If your children have not met your expectations, you may have strong feelings about this that you are holding inside your body. These can be particularly difficult to cope with because we are taught that there is something wrong with us if we have such feelings. But please remember that the feelings you hold inside your body for any reason can turn into physical problems that affect your health. Let yourself feel the truth of your own feelings, then record them in your journal.

Exercise 11

Being Unwanted

If you were the child of an unwanted pregnancy, you have got to have some feelings about it. Let yourself experience these. Take some time to write out how life has been for you and how you feel about that.

CHAPTER 10

Women and Their Pain

Suddenly I find myself churning inside like a troubled sea.

—NATALIE ROGERS

A woman in her early forties who was suffering from extreme fatigue came to me recently for healing. She was married and had a two-year-old child, and she was a supervisor in a large corporation. Although she loved her job, her husband, and her child, her life was extremely hectic. She had a difficult time asking for help, including the help of her husband. She was raised with the same beliefs that many of us were: It's the woman's job to do the cleaning, the cooking, and the laundry, to raise the children and still try to be attractive at the end of the day. Added to this, many women today work a nine-to-five job. My client told me she felt guilty when she complained about her life because it was all "really very nice."

When I channeled healing energy to her, she would cry and cry. Her body felt very sad about all that was expected of her each day. Her body really wanted a break!

Her medical doctors finally discovered that she had mononucleosis and told her that she was not to work for quite some time. I believe that her illness was her body's only way of getting her to slow down and make some changes in her life. She continued to come for healings, and it became increasingly obvious that she needed to change some of her attitudes and beliefs about herself and what was expected of her.

She learned to delegate some of her responsibilities. She learned to say no when she felt stretched to the limit. She accepted that she had limitations, which was really difficult for her to do. She looked at her physical problem in a holistic way. What was the mononucleosis about? What did it mean mentally, emotionally and spiritually, as well as physically? She made some tremendous changes because she was open to them and to the necessary healing. She healed rather quickly.

What It Means To Be A Woman

Let's look at what being a woman means to you. First of all, do you like being a woman? Do you like the way your life is? Are you happy with your role as a woman in general?

Are you a mother? Do you have a full-time job? Do you go to school? Are you in a relationship? Do you care for your parents or members of your family other than your children? Do you have a lot of responsibility? Do you ask for help when you need it? Are you the person you always wanted to be, or are you living the way others would like you to live?

There is a great deal of pressure right now on both men and women. It seems that in the last few years I am finding more and more women caught up in "superwoman" roles.

I worry about what all of that stress is doing to their bodies, especially when it is coupled with unresolved issues and the emotions surrounding them. Many women are angry about their treatment by society in general—and by co-workers, family members, and even other women. I've seen several women with mononucleosis, lupus, chronic fatigue syndrome, and clinical depression. Every one of them has a very difficult schedule, juggling school, kids, a full-time career, a relationship, or all of the above. They all knew before getting sick that they should slow down, make changes in their lives, delegate some of their responsibilities. But they just kept pushing themselves until they became physically sick.

Over the last few years I have also seen many women who are having trouble getting pregnant. One woman in her thirties was a very busy professional. She was also in school finishing her postgraduate studies. She and her new husband had just purchased a home, a fixer-upper, and were trying to get pregnant but with no luck.

I remember psychically looking inside her body, trying to get some information that would help with her inability to conceive. Her body said to me:

No way! I will not get pregnant. I'm already exhausted. I can only handle so much and right now I'm stressed to the limit with tight schedules and heavy demands on me. Tell her I will get pregnant only when there is a change in our lifestyle and I'm not expected to do so much all the time.

Her body also shared its fear concerning her husband's ambivalence about being a parent. She was afraid she might have to do all the parenting herself. Her body said there was a great deal to be figured out and changed before it would open itself up to a baby.

It is my belief that many of the health challenges women are having today are directly related to their role as women. For this reason it is more important than ever to take a very close look at our expectations for ourselves, what others are expecting of us, and how these expectations may be causing us some physical problems.

It's very difficult for many women to say no, to put themselves at the top of their own priority lists. It's difficult for them to delegate responsibilities to others, or to accept limitations. It is difficult for them to receive rather than always be giving.

Perhaps one of the most difficult areas for women to resolve and to integrate into their lives in a healthy way is their sexuality. Recently, I did two very intense hour-and-a-half healings on a woman who wanted her negative issues around sexuality to be healed. I have done several healings over the years for women who are struggling with being sexual. Usually these issues manifest themselves physically through the following:

ovulation problems

PMS (premenstrual syndrome)

difficult menstrual periods

fibroid cysts in the breasts

vaginal infections

ovarian and uterine cysts

fibroid tumors

herpes

cancer

difficult menopause

When I psychically looked at this particular woman's body, her negative attitudes, beliefs, and feelings were in her breasts. I saw images of past lives in which she bound up her breasts to hide them. There were feelings of shame around being a woman. She said that in this life she would often wear a very restricting bra to make her look smaller. She was trying to hide her femaleness.

John said that her negative attitudes and beliefs around her sexuality, her femaleness, her wants and desires as a woman, her sexual needs, were all issues she came into this lifetime to heal. I could feel the energy healing past-life pain. She cried a lot during our sessions. Many past-life images came to her as I channeled the energy.

It was an incredible healing! She said she felt that if she hadn't gotten the healings, along with working on her emotional issues with her therapist, that she would have gotten breast cancer. She said that ever since her breasts began to develop, she could feel an inner tenseness about them. It was as if she wished that they weren't there.

I have also seen numerous women struggle with their lack of sexual desires, such as a fifty-two-year-old woman who came in for healings of a recurring bladder problem. She told me that her husband really got on her nerves. She always felt angry with him. She didn't want to have sex with him, but didn't want to appear frigid either. So her body created a monthly bladder problem. This condition had continued for more than one year.

The pay-off was that her husband not only didn't ask her to have sex but was nice to her each time that she got another infection. For her healings to be complete, she had to address the issues she had with her husband by talking them out. If the bladder healed without resolving their conflicts, the emotional root of their issues would manifest in some other physical way. But she refused to talk with her husband about what was happening to her inside! She chose to keep the bladder problems rather than to look at her issues with her husband. Besides, there was the pay-off of his being nice to her whenever the bladder became infected. She simply refused to go to the root of her problem.

As a woman, it is easy for me to identify with others' struggles around their sexuality. I believe that all the sexual abuse I experienced as a child, the double messages I got about sex, and my not wanting to be a woman were the emotional roots for most of my female problems. I know I'm not alone in these beliefs because of all the women that I have seen over the years with the same or similar issues. They are women who don't want to be sexual, so their bodies create some kind of vaginal problem to use as an excuse, rather than to hurt their partner's feelings by saying no to their sexual advances. They are women who have guilt about enjoying themselves sexually or who are not married and feel guilty about having sex. Their bodies create vaginal problems as a form of punishment.

Looking at all our issues around sex can really be tough. I had been in therapy on and off for years, had talked about my confusion around sex, had talked about the sexual abuse with the babysitter. But until I was in my thirties I never really felt my anger or rage or sadness around these experiences. When I was 29, I went into surgically induced menopause after having a total hysterectomy. Both my ovaries, my fallopian tubes, my uterus, and my cervix were covered with benign tumors.

Today, I know that my reproductive organs had stored all of my feelings of rage, anger, sadness, hopelessness, resentment, and self-pity around being a woman and being abused, for some twenty years. These unresolved feelings turned into benign tumors. I think my body was saying, "I can't or don't want to be a dumping ground for all of these negative feelings anymore."

Shortly after the hysterectomy, I went into a severe depression and suffered from several physical and emotional symptoms, which I later discovered were menopause: hot flashes, nervousness, paranoia, anxiety, forgetfulness, and insomnia. Until I was put on the correct dosage of hormone replacement, every day was a nightmare. This actually turned out to be a blessing in disguise because I went back into therapy and really began looking at all of my issues around my sexuality and being a woman.

Most women I have known or done healings for have found it difficult to look at their feelings about being a woman. Are you having any recurring female problems, that is, trouble with any area of your body which identifies you as a woman or which has anything to do with your sexuality? Can you identify your feelings about being sexual? Perhaps going back to "Negative Feelings and Beliefs" (Chapter 3) will help you identify them. You'll have an opportunity to do more on this in the journal work section at the end of this chapter.

I had a client who hated her ex-husband. She told me he was into a lot of kinky sex and that when they were married having intercourse with him always disgusted her. She felt that it was her duty to have sex with him, so she never said no. Even though they had been divorced for a few years, she suffered from a lot of pain inside her vagina. It was very red, swollen, and constantly itched.

John said that this woman needed to forgive her ex-husband and herself. She was just as angry at herself for not saying no as she was towards her ex-husband for wanting kinky sex. Her healing process was long and painful. She cried on and off for weeks, which was very necessary. As we were healing layers of memories, other memories from her childhood surfaced. She had blocked out sexual abuse by her grandfather. This also needed to be healed.

Wake-Up Calls

If you are a woman and don't like it, if you are having difficulty with your role as a woman, or if you are having difficulty with your sexuality, you have suffered long enough. It's time to start healing. It's time to get free from this pain. The process will probably not be any more painful than the pain with which you already live. And once you have gone through it, you'll be free of it. The pain will end.

You deserve a happy, productive, stress-free, joy-filled life—not because of how hard you work or how good you look. You deserve it just because you are you. It is your birthright.

My belief now is that, as women, we are fortunate. We can find ways to have it all—all meaning anything we want—career, family, creativity, education, our own income, our own spirituality, rewarding friendships, fulfilling relationships. . . . The list goes on and on. Society's attitude, in general, is changing towards women. More and more doors open for us each day. But we can't have it all if we don't feel good.

JOURNAL WORK

The journal work which follows is designed to help you get in touch with feelings, attitudes, beliefs, and perhaps some unresolved issues that may be blocking you from having the kind of life you'd like to have.

Exercise 1
Your Feelings About Being a Woman

In your journal, write out your feelings about being a woman. It can be most helpful to go back to the list in Chapter 3 on "Negative Feelings and Beliefs." Write down what you feel about women in general and about your own role as a woman. What expectations do you have as a woman? Write down everything that comes to mind, allowing yourself to free-associate as you do.

* * *

Before going on to the next exercise, take a break. Put the book down and do something light. When you're ready, come back and go on to Exercise 2.

Exercise 2
Sexuality

Part A
Look at your feelings around your sexuality. Are you sexually active? How do you feel about it? Are you not sexually active? How do you feel about that?

Record your responses in your journal.

Part B
Ask yourself if there are any parts of your body that are feeling fearful or tense right now. Write those down and describe what you are experiencing.

Part C
Are there any questions you are hoping I won't ask? What are they and why are you hoping I won't ask?

Exercise 3
Connections Between Feelings and Physical Problems

Do you see any connection between your attitudes and beliefs about being a woman, your sexuality, and any physical problems you may be having? Please write these down in your journal.

When you're done with this journal entry, take another break.

Exercise 4
Inner Child Work

Part A

Put your pencil or pen in your nondominant hand and ask your inner child how she feels about being female. Record what she is feeling or saying to you.

Part B

Ask your inner girl how she feels about sex. Ask her what she would like to say about sex. Remember, her answers may be very different from your adult answers. Be patient with her. Give her all the time she needs to express herself. She may not know what to say. Make whatever she says okay. Remind her that she is safe and that you will protect her.

Part C

For a moment, give your critical parent an opportunity to say what she has to say. Write out her comments in your journal.

Exercise 5
Positive Womanhood

Once I became honest with myself and my therapist about the rage I felt, and began releasing the negative and hurtful feelings I had around being a woman and being sexual, I began to heal. I began to see the positive aspects of being a woman. We are beautiful, creative, spontaneous, passionate, loving, nurturing, playful, delightful human beings. I wouldn't trade places with anyone!

Part A

Write down in your journal your positive feelings and beliefs about being a woman. If you don't presently have any, move on to Part B.

Part B

Write down what you hope you will one day feel about being a woman.

CHAPTER 11

Men and Their Pain

When a man's self is hidden from everybody else . . . it seems also to become much hidden even from himself, and it permits disease and death to gnaw into his substance without his clear knowledge.

—Sidney Jourard

As a spiritual healer, I worry about men and their health. I see them as the real victims in our society from the standpoint that our society discourages them from expressing their emotions. I worry about the long-term effect this will have on their health.

Because men aren't given permission to express their feelings, they begin storing their pain at a very early age. When I psychically look inside men to see what's going on, I find that their bodies aren't as easy to read as are the bodies of women. I believe this is because men store so much deep inside.

I watch the boys playing in my neighborhood, and I have noticed that at a very early age they ridicule each other if they show any signs of pain, such as crying, when they are hurt.

Oftentimes, I will be working on a male client and see images of painful experiences inside them. But the men are usually so detached from their emotional memories and pain that they can't connect with the images I see.

As I mentioned earlier, I had a male client who came for healings of his asthma. When I placed my hands over his lungs, the image came to me of his father walking out the front door of his home when my client was three years old, never to return again. The child came down with asthma within a week of his father's leaving; moreover, he still suffers from it today! The spirit guides told me that this man had a serious abandonment issue, and it was sitting in his lungs, still affecting his health and relationships some thirty years later. The man told me that he had dealt with his father's leaving a long time ago and didn't believe it was affecting his health today. But I thought it was very interesting that the whole picture was still sitting in his lungs—and he was still suffering from asthma.

The Hazards of Being Male by Dr. Herb Goldberg was a difficult book for me to read because it really made me aware of the pain men experience. The more I read, the more upset I became. The author says, "Today one great difference between men and women is that women at least know they are oppressed." (p. i) I would love to quote the entire book for you, but since that's not possible I'm going to highly recommend that you read this book—whether you're a man or a woman.

Dr. Goldberg has a chapter in this book called "Impossible Binds," which says:

> *The male in our culture finds himself in countless "damned if you do, damned if you don't" no-win binds. He is constantly being affected by gross inconsistencies—between what he had been taught was "masculine" behavior as a boy and what is expected of him as an adult; between inner needs and social pressures; and between contradictory expectations in the many roles he has to play. He is psychologically fragmented by these many contradictory demands.*

Goldberg goes on to say that for survival's sake, most men are literally forced into being emotionally detached and out of touch with feelings of any kind. He states that:

> *The traditional male facade cool, detached, controlled, guarded, and disengaged—is a protective mechanism that allows him to respond simply to external cues or inputs, like a programmed computer, rather than having to wrestle with constant conflict and ambiguity.*
>
> *The first step in coping with this phenomenon is open recognition and acknowledgment of these binds. (p. 86).*

Dr. Goldberg describes many different binds that affect men's lives. One of the most devastating, in terms of our present discussion, is what he calls the "feeling bind." He points out that throughout life the male who expresses his feelings openly, or who "readily cries, screams, behaves sensually, etc.," learns that he may be looked upon as neurotic or unstable. By controlling his feelings, as he is expected to do, he "will inevitably become guarded, hidden, and emotionally unknown to himself and others and viewed as 'cold' and even hostile." Either way the man ends up losing. If he lets it all hang out, he is viewed as immature or "unmanly," lacking self-control. But if he holds in his emotions he is accused of being secretive, unemotional, and "overly self-controlled."

Dr. Goldberg goes on to say that a man can be released from impossible binds by reclaiming the deep feelings that lie hidden behind his defenses, recognizing and accepting them as part of himself. He may see them as a threatening part of himself, but at least he can then be in a position to choose whether or not he is going to risk being true to the real self behind his defenses. Dr. Goldberg points out:

> *Undoubtedly, the re-owning of the real self will precipitate a crisis in the lives of all men who have allowed themselves to be bound up in these annihilating conflicts. It may therefore be necessary to acknowledge the need for help with these struggles and to seek it from a competent therapist. (p. 97)*

Men have gotten so many mixed messages over the years. They are told to get their anger out, yet are reminded not to lose their tempers. They need to express their feelings more, yet we give them another message that says, "Don't be too emotional because that is a sign of weakness." We want them to be more sensitive. More romantic. More sentimental. On the other hand, we say, "Go off to war and protect us. Kill whoever you have to, just don't come back and tell us about it. Come back and be the loving, sensitive, trusting, romantic guy you were before you left."

If you are a man, mixed messages can be causing you many physical problems, as well as emotional ones. Dr. Goldberg's book reveals a lot about the source of men's pain, but what is most disturbing is that most men don't know they're in pain nor why. Men have learned to deny their feelings, wants, desires, needs, and physical pain. They are always supposed to strive harder, compete, and yet be nice guys. They don't know how to reach out to friends because they are taught at an early age to compete with each other. When they do socialize, the conversations are not deep and elaborate but tend to be superficial. They learn to avoid topics that would make them appear needy. As Dr. Goldberg points out, a man's inner life is filled with lessons that put him in emotional double-binds or impossible-binds and leave him lonely and in despair.

Another story comes to mind of a man who came to me for healings involving his diabetes. There were images inside his pancreas of a great deal of shame around his leaving the Seventh-Day Adventist church in which he had been raised. He said to me:

> *The impact of joining the SDA church saturated every facet of my life. Suddenly, we were very active churchgoers. We went to church at least four to five times per week; we studied daily Sabbath school lessons; we became vegetarians, and we were active in church missions and associated primarily with church members. There were shames for not being more holy, and we were entreated to be more obedient or we would go to hell. There was immense guilt for breaking any of the rules.*

When he turned twenty-five, he decided to leave the church against his family's wishes. Within weeks, he came down with diabetes. He has been coming for healings for close to five years now. He has had to work on layers and layers of shame about his decision to go against the family and the church. He's had a struggle with his relationship with God, because for a long time he truly believed God had given him the disease of diabetes as punishment.

His issues around sexuality have surfaced. His codependency has become apparent to him, too. He is always being "Mr. Nice Guy," saying yes to everyone so the boat doesn't get rocked or anyone upset. He's had to learn that it's okay to do and be what feels right for him in spite of what any others want or need him to do. He has worked on several issues that have slowly surfaced, one by one, during our healing sessions.

He decided to seek therapy to aid him in his healing work. The healings bring up issues, memories, past pain, and his therapist helps him to heal from these emotionally. It's been fascinating to watch the process of a wonderful combination of spiritual and emotional healing. He is so much happier today and feels more whole.

I see so many men struggle for their freedom from the roles and expectations society has put on them. Many men choose to go along with what's expected of them rather than go through the hassle of challenging the status quo. They avoid making major changes because it seems easier that way. But again, consider the price for this in terms of their health!

In my opinion, many of the heart attacks men suffer are broken hearts—literally the injured hearts of people who never lived the way they wanted to. They got caught up in doing what was expected of them.

No doubt the most challenging and harmful expectation we place on men is sending them off to war, to "serve their country." I've seen several men who served in Vietnam; one client comes to mind. He is a man in his early forties with bad knees and chronic back, neck, and shoulder problems. When I looked inside, I saw memories of Vietnam: hate, rage, sadness that he had to go, and for all that he saw and had to do. Resentment for losing four years of his youth. I asked him if he cried or yelled out his feelings. He replied, "What good would it do?"

A great line in the movie *Prince of Tides* occurred when the psychiatrist asked the brother of his patient, "Did you ever cry over your brother's death"?

"What good would it do; it wouldn't bring him back," he said.

The psychiatrist replied, "No, but it might bring you back!"

I see so many men full of old pain, old memories, old injustices done to them. But for some reason or other, they don't want to go inside and get that stuff out of there. Many don't believe the past can affect them as much as it does. Many struggle with the idea that unresolved issues could be sitting inside their bodies, preferring not to believe that such a thing might be possible.

I believe that one saving grace for men is all their physical activity. Exercise can work a lot of old pain out of the body, but I also believe that if some really serious issues are in there, issues such as sexual, physical, or emotional abuse, they need to be talked out with a competent therapist and dealt with. If not, they will forever affect all current and future relationships with co-workers, significant others, children—and themselves!

Lazaris, an entity who channels information through Jach Pursel, says, "Remember to use Vietnam as a tool, not as your destroyer." (*Body, Mind, and Spirit,* October 1989). For many, Vietnam will be their destroyer. Still, now . . . twenty years later, if you are full of pain, full of hurt, full of painful memories, full of hate and sadness, those feelings will kill you in one way or another. Get the war out of there.

You already served your time. You do not need to continue to be in bondage to the Vietnam War! Find yourself a good veterans support group and talk. Then talk some more until it all comes out. If you need to yell, then yell! Do whatever you need to do to be *free*! Doesn't that sound good? Free? As I said, you served your time; you don't need to carry it around with you anymore. But, chances are, you'll need some help getting Nam out of you. Please don't let pride get in your way! It's not worth it, either now or in the long run. Consider the following quote from Sidney Jourard's book, *The Transparent Self*:

> *When a man's self is hidden from everybody else . . . it seems also to become much hidden even from himself, and it permits disease and death to gnaw into his substance without his clear knowledge.*

Men don't listen to the warning signals that their bodies send out when something is wrong. (Women aren't very good at it either.) They deny physical or emotional pain because it's not "manly." They go to work when they don't feel well because they hate appearing helpless or dependent. Staying in bed because of sickness is the only acceptable way they can pamper themselves—but many won't even do that.

Men pride themselves on not missing any time at work, which is another reason they don't pay attention to those early warning signals from their bodies. They have a tendency to prove that they can resist, ignore, and overcome signs of illness.

We all—men and women—need to be more sensitive to our bodies, to listen to our dreams and be true to ourselves.

Get rid of the layers of other people's stuff that are on you: your mom's, your dad's, your partner's, your children's, your boss's, everybody else's expectations. Peel away those layers of other people's wants, needs, and desires for you. Get down to your own. You are in there somewhere! Please, give yourself a chance to survive the hazards of being male. Only you can free yourself from the internal pain that is common to most men. Without hurting yourself or anyone else, do whatever you've got to do to begin to be free . . . then keep going!

JOURNAL WORK

Exercise 1

An Inventory of Fundamental Needs

Go over the following list of questions, answering each one as honestly as possible. As you go along, record in your journal any thoughts, ideas, or feelings that come up.

1. Do you feel your feelings?
2. Do you get nurturing from others?
3. Can you take care of yourself emotionally? Physically?
4. Can you cry? Do you?
5. Do you ask for what you need?
6. Do you know what you need?
7. Do you know and have conversations with the kind of people you would like to?
8. Do you have friendships with other men?
9. Are they satisfying for you?
10. What do you do when you feel sad?
11. Who protects you?
12. Who was or is your hero? Why?
13. What are your burdens?
14. What do you do when you feel angry? Enraged?
15. What do you do when you are physically hurt?
16. Do you ask for help when you need it?
17. What do you do when you make a mistake?
18. How do you feel when you make a mistake?
19. What do you expect from other men, in general?

20. Have you ever lost a family member or close friend? How did you deal with the loss?
21. Are you happy with your sexuality?
22. Are you the kind of sexual partner you want to be?
23. Do you express yourself sexually?
24. Do you allow yourself to express your passion?
25. How do you express your creativity?
26. Do you have a hobby?
27. Do you ever let your imagination flow?
28. Do you have a lot of pride? Where does it show up?
29. What limitations do you feel as far as being a man?
30. When was the last time someone held you? Comforted you?
31. When was the last time someone bought you a present?
32. Do you ever worry about losing control?
33. What do you think would happen if you let go of feelings such as: Sadness? Anger? Frustration? Guilt? Shame?
34. Has your heart ever been broken? What did you do with the feelings you had? What did you do with your feelings of loss?
35. Did you allow yourself to feel the pain or did you try to replace the feelings of loss with something else?
36. What about your body? Does it look the way you'd like it to?
37. Do you have an image of the way you are supposed to look?
38. How do you express your joy?
39. Do you feel responsible for other people? Who? How come?
40. What regrets do you have?
41. What makes you feel guilty?
42. Do you respect yourself?
43. Do people take you seriously?

44. Do you take yourself seriously?
45. What is weakness to you?
46. What do you do when you watch a sad movie?
47. As a child, what were the messages you received from adult males in your life about being a man?
48. As a child, what were the messages you received from adult women in your life about being a man? Their expectations?
49. What is it like for you to be a man?
50. What would you like to change about yourself or your life?

Notice that there are no "right" or "wrong" answers here. These are questions that each person will answer in his own way.

Exercise 2
The Little Boy Within

With your nondominant hand, ask your little boy inside what it's been like for him to be a boy. Then ask him to write down what it has been like for him to be a man.

Exercise 3
War Experiences

One of the most difficult experiences a person can face is having to go to war. While many men consider it a man's duty to "serve his country" in this way, it is nevertheless inevitable that they will have strong feelings about it once they get out. If you are a Vietnam veteran, or the veteran of any armed conflict, take this opportunity to get in touch with what the experience meant for you.

Part A
Record in your journal any memories or feelings that come up for you around serving your country in an armed conflict.

Part B
If you did not serve in Vietnam or other armed conflict, you may still have feelings about it. Write them down in your journal.

CHAPTER 12

Unfinished Business

As we change, our relationships change, but whatever form they take, they can serve as mirrors of unacknowledged parts of ourselves.

—FRANCES VAUGHAN

Someone once told me that relationships are tools for us to learn about ourselves. I didn't want to hear that! Relationships are *supposed* to be about love and romance. You grow up. You meet Mr. or Ms. Right. You fall in love, get married, and the two of you live happily ever after. Falling in love can be the most powerful experience there is. It seems to hold so many promises of the good in life. Somehow, when we're in love we believe that we'll never experience the feelings of loneliness, abandonment, fear, despair, and hopelessness again.

I hate to bring up my own past relationships. They all started out with a bang—that exhilarating feeling of being in love—only to quickly become painfully difficult. For so many years, I did not know how to have a healthy relationship. I didn't know what I wanted other than to be happy. Unfortunately, I didn't know what happiness was. One man to whom I was engaged *beat me up only a little.* At that time, this was happiness in comparison to another man I had previously dated who loved to bounce me off the walls.

Once I started becoming healthy, I realized that getting hit or being beat up was not happiness, nor was it healthy, nor was it something that I deserved or wanted. Each man was a little bit healthier than the previous one. Once I identified what physical abuse was, I moved on to emotional abuse. That was tougher to see because of my many beliefs about myself:

I am unworthy	I am worthless
I am unwanted	I am unlovable
I am a victim	I am abandoned
I am betrayed	I am no good
I am unattractive	I am incapable
I am undeserving	I am a burden
I am inadequate	I am inferior
I am sinful	I deserve pain
Life is meant to be hard!	

The emotionally abusive men I associated with also had similar beliefs about themselves. I seemed to attract men who also didn't know how to have healthy relationships. Together, we fumbled our way through, always with the shared hope of making it work. My own negative beliefs kept me going in a seemingly endless circle of painful relationships. Surprisingly, some of them were somewhat satisfying, enough to keep me there. It has taken years of unraveling my stored feelings and healing my beliefs for me to have the kind of satisfying and loving relationships I have today.

For a long time, the problem was that I would get out of one and into another without really healing the hurt. I would take all of the feelings and reinforced negative beliefs into the next relationship.

I had some big issues around abandonment. I was so afraid that no one would love me. When someone did, I feared that they would leave me. My fears of abandonment really brought out my codependent behavior. I would always do my best to make sure that the man in my life needed me. I figured as long as I was needed I would not be abandoned.

It wasn't until I got into recovery that I became aware of my dependency on men. My sponsor told me to stay away from men for two years and get to know myself. He told me that I really needed to do some serious work on myself if I ever wished to be happy in love. He helped me realize that I wasn't free.

Slowly I discovered that my fears of abandonment controlled all my relationships. I had to look at layers and layers of issues, beliefs and feelings around men and dependency. Behind this dependency was a whole storehouse of old feelings, including worthlessness, shame, fear, hatred, anger, rage, bitterness, disappointment, etc. It is so important for us to heal our hearts from the pain of the past, in order to make room for love—both for now and in the future!

I recently saw my ex-husband after not seeing him for two years. We were in therapy a lot during our four-year marriage. I had dealt with much of the anger and rage I felt about certain things that had taken place, so I was amazed at how much anger and resentment were still inside me! I really thought that I had released my feelings until I saw him face-to-face and discovered otherwise.

Memories started welling up from within my body, memories that I had all but forgotten. Along with the memories came feelings that I didn't want to feel. I didn't want to deal with those feelings. I had hoped that maybe they would just go away. Within twenty-four hours, I had pain in my jaw. I didn't want to believe that it had anything to do with my ex-husband, but I knew that my body was talking to me.

I turned to Louise Hay's book, *Heal Your Body.* In it she says that jaw problems have to do with "anger, resentments, desire for revenge." That's exactly how I was feeling, everything she named helped to explain the feelings I had toward my ex-husband. I didn't want to feel this way, but I could not deny the truth of my feelings. I had to own up to them. It was as if my jaw were saying, "Don't hold this anger in. Get it out. Don't tighten up and keep the words in."

The next stage in this healing process occurred a couple days later, before I was to see him again. He was coming to our home to pick up some things he had left behind. My hip developed a very strange pain. Again I turned to Louise Hay's book. It told me that hip problems are "fear of moving forward in major decisions, or nothing to move forward to."

Where that fits in is that my ex-husband was going to take part of our furniture and other things around the house that had been a part of my life for six years. I didn't want to go through that experience. I wanted everything to stay just the way it was. After all the decisions had been made about who was going to take what, the pain in my hip stopped.

Next, I needed to get my feelings out. I did not want to store those old feelings inside any longer. I asked God for the courage to say what I needed to say and to help me with my choice of words. A small voice inside kept saying, "Don't rock the boat; just stay mellow; you can work this stuff out on your own; it's not that big a deal, anyway."

Fortunately, the words did come out, along with the anger, the hurt, and my frustration. I said everything that I needed to say. I was fortunate because my ex-husband was willing to listen to it all. I yelled. I cried. I was so angry that our marriage hadn't worked. It took me a couple of days to work through the process of releasing my ex-husband, my marriage, and all of my dreams about marriage. Even though I had cried on and off prior to and after our divorce, there was still more sadness, anger, resentment and bitterness. I wanted the process to happen overnight, but it took time.

Truly, relationships often do seem to mirror back to us who we are. If we are close to another person, the feelings we are holding in our bodies will affect how we relate to each other. We may see reflected in the other person those things that we haven't allowed ourselves to see in ourselves. Or our own hidden feelings of being unworthy may attract us to people who will treat us as unworthy or even be abusive to us. Similarly, if we are carrying around a lot of resentment, anger, or rage, we may be attracted to people whose own low self-esteem draws them to us, triggering our own abusiveness.

By going inside and asking what is being mirrored back to us by a relationship, we get in touch with the stored feelings we have been unable or unwilling to look at. Healing starts when, instead of blaming the other person for our pain, we look inside ourselves at the pain that is already there. This does not mean taking the blame for the other person's behavior. And it doesn't mean that it is okay to allow the other person to continue to be abusive to us. But only by healing the feelings that bring us together can we truly be free to choose the kinds of relationships we want.

Shakti Gawain talks about relationships as mirrors. What she says really made a difference for me in my perception of my relationships:

> *I assume that everything in my life is my reflection, my creation; there are no accidents or events that are unrelated to me. If I see or feel something, if it has any impact on me, then my being has attracted or created it to show me something. If it didn't mirror some part of myself, I wouldn't even be able to see it. All of the people in my life are reflections of the various characters and feelings that live inside of me. (*Living in the Light, *p. 26).*

I am still learning how to interpret the reflections of myself in others. This has taught me a lot about myself. Here are some examples of how this mirroring process has worked in my life:

Example:
I used to feel that my ex-husband didn't pay enough attention to me.

Deep down inside, however, I believed that I didn't deserve a lot of attention unless I was doing something for someone. I couldn't handle a lot of attention. It made me feel uncomfortable. Realistically, the amount of attention my husband paid me was exactly what I was comfortable with, even though I thought that I wanted more.

Example:
I used to feel as though I did all of the work in the relationship and around the house, and I resented it.

My belief was that it was my job to do all of the work in the relationship and around the house. It was the job of the woman of the house to keep everything running smoothly. That's a nice coverup for me wanting to control everything. Realistically, I needed a man who was willing to let me do all of the work in the home and for the relationship.

Example:
An old boyfriend used to criticize my body, my weight, my appearance. I was never good enough.

My belief was that, indeed, I was not good enough. I was constantly picking on my body, weight, and appearance. I never felt adequate. Realistically, I needed a man who reflected my discontent with myself. I could handle that. Back then, I could have never handled a man who accepted me for who and what I was.

Example:
Throughout most of my relationships, I have felt cheated because I didn't feel that I was getting all of the love and nurturing I wanted and needed.

My belief was that I didn't deserve any more than I was getting. I could handle small amounts. It didn't embarrass me or make me feel obligated to them. It felt too suffocating to get any more.

* * *

As my beliefs have changed, so have my relationships. Five years ago, I wouldn't have been able to be with the man I am with today. I wouldn't have felt worthy of his acceptance, loving tenderness or nurturing. Learning to be in a relationship has certainly been a process for me. I continually learn about myself.

What is he reflecting back about me? If I think that he is being critical, is he reflecting my criticism? Yes! When I get upset because I don't like the way he takes care of himself, is that a reflection of how poorly I am taking care of myself? Yes! If I get upset with him for not expressing his feelings more, is it really I who doesn't express my feelings? Yes. Mirrors everywhere.

It brings us back to my statement at the beginning of this chapter, that relationships are tools for us to learn about ourselves. If you are in a relationship, give this mirror concept a try. Learn more about yourself. If you're not in a relationship and would like to be, I'd like to recommend two things:

First, do the journal work at the end of this chapter to make sure you are not going to carry old pain into your next relationship. Perhaps the reason you're not in a relationship now is because there's no room in your heart for new love until you get the memories of old relationships out of there.

Second, look at your beliefs about love and what you deserve. You might find that some beliefs that you are holding inside are that you don't deserve to have happiness, or that love is too painful, or that you don't feel worthy of the love you need. Examine those beliefs! As unromantic as this statement may be, relationships are tools for us to learn about ourselves. Of course, they can also be wonderful, loving, nurturing, and full of joy, and ultimately that's what we want from them.

We do create our own realities—a process that begins with what we believe. If you want to change the nature and the quality of your relationships and your life, begin by changing your beliefs about yourself and what you deserve.

Sexually Transmitted Diseases

An important area of unfinished business that sometimes comes up around relationships has to do with sexually transmitted diseases: syphilis, gonorrhea, scabies, lice, candidiasis, vaginal infections such as trichomoniasis and chlamydia, nonspecific urethritis, venereal warts, herpes, and AIDS. All of these diseases are physically painful and emotionally scarring. With these diseases we often experience shame, embarrassment, fear, hopelessness, powerlessness, anger, terror, rage, feelings of doom, disgust, sadness, guilt, desperation, isolation, panic, regret, remorse, resentment, feeling used, betrayed, sinful, abused, bitter, anxious, hateful, helpless, lonely, hostile, suicidal, overwhelmed, exposed. All of these feelings can arise when we are infected with a sexually transmitted disease.

Frequently we don't know what to do with our feelings when we find out that we've been infected, especially by someone we love and have trusted. So we usually internalize all our feelings and hope they will go away, just as the disease's symptoms slowly fade away with medication. People with herpes and AIDS, however, aren't so lucky, since at the present time we don't have any cures for them.

For those of you who do have a sexually transmitted disease that cannot be cured with medication, you've got to have a lot of feelings about this injustice. If you've had to deal with a sexually transmitted disease, either in the past or present, exercises in the journal section will help you address all of your feelings around what you went through or are going through. It is very important in your healing process to get all of those feelings out of your body!

JOURNAL WORK

Exercise 1

Naming Names

Before you begin, turn to a clean page in your journal and draw a vertical line an inch or two from the left margin. You will end up with two separate columns, narrow on the left, wide on the right. Label the left column "Names," the right one, "Your unfinished emotional pain."

Sit comfortably. Take a few deep breaths and exhale slowly and gently. Close your eyes and ask your body, "Who's in there with whom I have unfinished business?" And what is the unfinished business?

A name may come. A face. An experience you may have forgotten. Don't just keep those names or images in your head. Write down the names and unfinished business here.

Exercise 2
Locating the Pain

Still in a relaxed state, write down any of the physical pain that you are feeling as a result of working on Exercise #1. Do certain parts or areas of your body hurt? Acknowledge that pain to yourself by describing it in your journal. Don't discount the physical pain that may come up as the result of looking at your love relationships. You will probably discover that the pained areas are where you are storing these feelings.

Exercise 3
Mirrors

Now take a look at what your love relationships are mirroring to you. If you need to, go back and review some of my mirrors I discussed previously. Perhaps that will help clarify what your own relationships are mirroring for you. Then record what you discover in your journal.

Exercise 4
Sexually Transmitted Diseases

Most people who have had to deal with a sexually transmitted disease have very strong feelings about it, which are often hidden from conscious awareness. If you have had such a disease, write down in your journal the feelings you have around what you went through or are still going through.

Exercise 5
Who Infected You?

Describe your feelings toward the person(s) who infected you, whether you know who they are or not.

Exercise 6
Others' Reactions

Write about how other people in your life reacted when they heard that you had contracted this disease. Were they fearful? Supportive? Sympathetic? Understanding? Or did they avoid or reject you? Did they criticize or abandon you?

Exercise 7
Your Feelings About Others' Reactions

Describe how you felt, or are still feeling, about other people's reactions as you described them in the previous exercise.

Exercise 8
What You Can Do

What can you do with the pain you have discovered in this chapter? Here are a few suggestions:

1. Talk it all over with your therapist.
2. Get your feelings out. Yell, scream, cry. Beat pillows. Do some rigorous exercise, without hurting yourself or others.
3. If you have a picture of the person who hurt you, tape it to the top of a chair. Pretend that this person is sitting in the chair and tell him or her everything you have ever wanted to tell them.
4. Write a letter to the person, which you don't have to mail. Say everything that you have wanted to tell them.
5. Ask a Higher Power, God, or the Universe, to show you how to heal this pain.
6. Get some healings on your heart or whatever other body part hurts.
7. Get a massage to help your body release these old feelings.
8. Most importantly, be willing to release this pain, the stories, and the resentments.

CHAPTER 13

Religion

Religion in its humility restores man to his only dignity, the courage to live by grace.
—George Santayana

This chapter has been difficult for me to write. Let me try to explain by sharing a story that Reverend Jim Fisher recently told in a sermon.

> *There was a little girl who always looked on the bright side of everything. No matter what was happening, she always looked for the good. Her brothers were really tired of her positiveness so they decided to play a trick on her. They filled the barn with manure and sent her down there to get something, hoping that she would get all dirty, stinky, and sad. The little girl was gone for quite some time, and her brothers started to worry. They thought that they had better go and see if she was okay. They walked into the barn and there she was, smiling and shoveling away! They asked her what she was doing, and she replied, "With all of this manure, there must be a pony in here somewhere!"*

It's a wonderful story, but Reverend Jim didn't end it there. He went on to say that, probably, if the little girl had expected a shark in there, she would have never dug down to find out. Then he went into his sermon about when we know, deep inside, that we are good and wonderful and loved, that we let our lights shine. We radiate our goodness and purity to the world. We know the goodness in us exists and, therefore, we look for it in others. The flip side of that is when we believe that we're bad, shameful sinners we want to cover ourselves up so people don't see how awful we feel. We lose our spontaneity. We don't express our joy because we don't feel joyful about who we are.

This is where my struggle comes in writing this chapter. I believe that many religions, or perhaps I should say church leaders, reinforce negative feelings and beliefs that we have about ourselves. I'm not saying all religions do this, but many of them do.

Being a psychic and a spiritual healer for twenty-five years has shown me a lot about the negativity of religions. I know about this negativity in two ways: first, through the clients I have worked with over the years; second, through the religious people who have never met me, yet believe that I am evil and what I do is evil. It's tough to turn the other cheek sometimes and allow others to have their opinions without getting into a debate.

Many religious people I have encountered love to talk about Satan. They go on and on about his powers. In a ten-minute conversation, they will mention Satan fifteen to twenty times and God once, if He's lucky! To me, it's all such a contradiction! They say they've got Jesus in their heart, yet they love to dwell on Satan. My parents taught me to pray for these people—to ask God to bless them. I have to admit, there have been many times when I have prayed for them and my heart wasn't in it!

I don't understand what gives people the right to judge others as evil or as sinners. Jesus did say "Judge them by their fruits," which I believe means that if you are going to judge people, judge them by their lives, by what they do with their gifts, their attitudes towards others, their whole essence. Get to know someone, then make your judgments based on what you have learned about them rather than on what you have heard or what you fear.

Many people believe that church has to be condemnatory and harsh, shameful, and punishing in order to be effective. They believe we all have to be put in our places and reminded that we are sinners, that we are fallen. I have seen some people come to the church that I belong to and really agonize over how positive it is. They don't believe they deserve it. Some people don't believe church is supposed to make you feel good.

Another thing that I have encountered as a spiritual healer is the whole idea people seem to have about their religion: "My religion, my belief, my church is the only true church and better than yours." Several stories of clients come to mind, and I'd like to share one with you because it has always stuck in my mind.

A man called one day for a healing on his heart. He'd had a very bad heart attack and was now recovering from it. His Charismatic wife was very anxious about me doing any healings on him because

I'm not a Charismatic. I did a healing on him one evening while his wife sat in a nearby chair, praying constantly, rocking back and forth. She was very nervous. She couldn't look at me. The healing energy was very strong that night. The man was crying and told me that he could really feel the presence of God working through my hands. When we were done, he told me that he wanted to see me for more healings. The next day he called to say that his wife had talked to their Charismatic priest who told her that, since I wasn't a Charismatic, I couldn't really channel God's energy and that I must be working for Satan!

The priest told her not to let her husband come back! According to my client, the priest had said to her, "It was obviously God's will that your husband have a heart attack and that he must learn to live with it." He told me that, as much as he believed in what I did, he couldn't upset his wife. So he was not coming back!

I don't want to give you the idea that I'm picking on Charismatics. I have had many people from many different religions tell me that because I didn't belong to their religion, I obviously wasn't channeling God's energy. When I hear this, I feel angry. Didn't Jesus say to the Corinthians, "These gifts I give unto you and greater works shall you do." He didn't go on to say, ". . . but only if you're a Catholic, an Episcopalian, or a Jew." He said, "You." That means me, you—all of us! No conditions. Simply, I give these gifts to you.

Until I began working on and healing my beliefs about myself, I could not have gone week after week to a church that preached what a wonderful child of God I was. For so long, I felt there was something really wrong with me and I was always afraid that people would be able to see all that bad stuff. It made me too uncomfortable to hear a lot of positive things about myself or to be told that, as a child of God, I had all the capabilities to do or be anything that I wanted. Yet, I have to admit, as Reverend Jim said, we know deep down at the core of our being that *we are good.* And that's probably why I kept digging for that pony in my life! I had to shovel away the manure and find the goodness.

To me, that's what religion should be doing for all of us. It should be encouraging us to shovel away our negative beliefs and feelings about ourselves, which we have acquired along the way. It should be helping us to discover our goodness. Our holiness. Our divinity. If we are created in God's image, wouldn't that mean we have unlimited potential? That we are made out of the good in God? If you are the son or daughter of the highest source in the Universe, you can't get much better!

Some readers are going to jump on that last statement right away! What about all of the evil people? The people who kill and abuse others? They, too, are children of God, but it's probably been lifetimes since anyone told them so. Their goodness is in there. It's just that, with all of the manure inside (negative beliefs about themselves), they probably don't even dare to look for fear they'll never find it! Their belief that they are bad is constantly reinforced by society, which includes many religions.

Do you ever feel an inner tug or conflict when someone brings up the word religion? Most of my conflict comes from the inner child *knowing* what is true about God and Jesus versus what the outer world says is true about God and Jesus. I have already shared with you a little about my adult struggles with religion. Now, here are my inner child's feelings on the subject:

Nothing brings such an inner feeling of joy and total contentment as when my inner child thinks and feels God. She has never seen God, yet she knows that God exists and totally loves her from the top of her head to the tip of her toes. God is like a warm, cuddly blanket. A huge bouquet of colorful balloons. A puppy or kitty. Just thinking about God and feeling God makes her smile all over! She says God is the best there is; God made me and loves me, and He wants me to be happy.

She says that God gets sad when we feel sad. God hears everything and loves to laugh with us. She says that God thinks she is the most precious person He ever made and then says that God says that about everyone, because we are all really special. We all have talents. We are each different. She says God's arms are "sooooo big that He can hug everyone at the same time." She says God never lets any of us down. Sometimes we can't hear what His answers are, but He always answers us.

My adult self asked her to tell me about Jesus. She beams from ear to ear. She squeals in delight. Jesus is her older brother, who came to earth a long time ago to teach us how to live our lives, so that we can be happy and others can be, too. She says that He gave us the Golden Rule and told us to live our lives accordingly. She says that He was wonderful and gentle and even though He is physically dead, He still lives in her memory, which is located in her heart. She says she loves it when we meditate, because then she can sit and feel herself in God's lap, feeling her oneness with everyone in the world. She does not understand why adults have made it all so complicated! Jesus said we need to "be as little children, in order to enter into the Kingdom of Heaven." I believe that's because, as children, we know in our hearts that we are good and that God is good. We know we deserve happiness.

As children, knowing the goodness in our hearts, we would have no trouble believing we deserve the Kingdom of Heaven. As adults, with all the "shoulds" and the conditions we place on love, it would be impossible to know in our hearts that we deserve the Kingdom of Heaven. All the voices of the world—parents, grandparents, co-workers, children, religious leaders, politicians, scientists, doctors, all the adults who have unresolved negative beliefs about themselves—will pass those beliefs onto others.

If we believe bad things about ourselves, we will find others to reinforce those beliefs until one day, that little pony inside makes enough noise to be heard. Then a voice from deep inside will say, "Hey, I'm good. I am loved. I am precious. I deserve the best in life God has provided for me."

Look honestly at the religious system you follow. Does it reinforce your goodness or does it reinforce those negative beliefs that you have about yourself? Are you constantly reminded about shortcomings? Are you told every week that you are a sinner? That you're bad? That you are fallen and you do not deserve happiness? What beliefs does your current religion reinforce? Can you be honest with yourself about this?

In your heart, you will know if you're good or not. You will know the truth about God. I remember hearing in a sermon that God told Moses, "My truth is written on your heart."

If you have discovered that your religion does reinforce your negative beliefs about yourself, it's important to start thinking about finding one that will reinforce your goodness. The problem here is that you need to start believing in it yourself. So what comes first—the chicken or the egg? It doesn't matter. What does matter is that this process of knowing your goodness begin now. Enough time has been wasted wallowing in the badness! Ask God to help direct you to a church or religion that will help you start to know about your goodness. I really believe in my heart that that's what God wants for you. He wants you to find that pony!

JOURNAL WORK

Exercise 1
Your Present Religion

Ask yourself if your present religion reinforces your essential goodness or if it reinforces negative beliefs you have about yourself. The reinforcement of the positive is important to your healing. If you are holding negative feelings about yourself inside your body, this cannot be a positive influence on your health.

Write down in your journal the kinds of beliefs your church reinforces and your feelings about these.

This exercise is important because religion plays a critical role in our lives. Even if you are an atheist, or haven't been to church in twenty years, old religious teachings from your childhood can still be affecting you.

Record your insights, your beliefs, your memories and your feelings about religion in your journal.

Exercise 2
How Your Religion Reinforces Parents' Teachings

Sometimes the negative beliefs we find in our church experiences reinforce or carry on negative beliefs or feelings that our parents taught us. Take the time to look at this possibility. If your parents were raised to believe in badness, the chances are they will raise you the same way. This cycle goes on and on until that tiny voice inside says, "Hey, I'm in here and I'm good because I was created by God!"

Exercise 3
Your Inner Child and Religion

Ask your inner child to describe God and any figures that are important in your religion. This can be done through words or with a drawing. Include in this any details about his/her relationship with God.

CHAPTER 14

The Weight Game

If you want to know the secret of good health, set up home in your own body, and start loving yourself when there.

— John W. Travis, M.D.

I was recently with a woman who is the sales manager for a well-known weight loss program. Since I have had a weight problem most of my life, it was very difficult for me to sit and listen to her rave about winning a cruise for having the highest sales. What struck me as I listened to her was that she talked about weight loss as a product, much as one would discuss cars or computers. The emotional aspects of being overweight were never mentioned; the discussion was reduced to sales and bonuses. It was a business, plain and simple. All of those overweight people were just figures in the books at the end of each month.

After years and years of dieting on my own, joining weight loss programs, working out at health clubs, buying workout tapes, taking diet pills, surviving on protein drinks, and reading all of the latest diet books, I have come to believe that food is only 25 percent of the reason we are overweight. Lack of exercise is another 25 percent. Fifty percent of why I am overweight is because of unresolved emotions. After years of picking on myself and being picked on for being overweight, I have come to realize that weight has served several purposes for me.

When I was little, food comforted me. I often felt lonely as a child and have fond memories of Twinkies filling that void. Oreo cookies helped when I felt afraid or sad. Many times, when I was little and hurt myself, someone gave me a cookie and it always made me feel better! Now, wanting to feel better is strongly associated with eating food.

I recently heard an advertisement on the radio for an eating disorders clinic in Minneapolis. It was a word association test in which the narrator, usually a therapist, said a word and the person taking the test said the first thing that came to mind. The commercial went something like this:

Narrator Word Association	*Client Response*
afraid	cookies
sad	ice cream
alone	pizza
mad	hot dogs
panic	potato chips
overwhelmed	doughnuts
anxious	Snickers candy bar
rage	licorice

This pushed some emotional buttons inside me. I felt fearful because these were my issues about food. It's always been difficult for me to express my feelings; it's much easier to stuff them down with food. This way only I suffer and the person I am angry with or afraid of does not.

Despite the billion-dollar weight loss industry in this country, we are not conquering our weight problem. How many times have you read in the paper about the ridiculously high percentage of people who lose weight, only to gain it back within the first year?

This is because food is serving a purpose other than nourishing our bodies. Weight is also serving a purpose!

The only problem is that few people or institutions are addressing the real issues.

Recently, I went through a weight loss program. I struggled each day to get rid of the walls of protection that I have put around myself. I changed my eating habits, learned to exercise more, kept a food journal, learned about nutrition and low-fat cooking, and how to grocery shop in a healthier way. It was all very helpful, but all the other weight loss programs teach the very same things. The only difference with this one was that it offered a support group. It was helpful to be a part of a group of people who were all dealing with their emotional issues around weight gain and loss. This group met weekly for eight weeks. Then the corporate office said it couldn't continue because they were afraid someone would sue them for pretending to be professional counselors. We had all been commenting that we believed these sessions were what was making the difference in our weight loss. This was a major letdown for all of us!

I have come to believe that being thin will not come from going on diets for the rest of my life. While people need to cut back on caloric intake to get those pounds off, they also must look at what the food does *for* them emotionally. This will enable them to keep the weight off. Whatever food did for me as a kid, it's doing for me as an adult. This realization led me to ask myself: What is my behavior around food? When do I turn to it? No matter what time of day it is, if I feel empty, lonely, afraid, sad, angry, overwhelmed, or anxious, food is my comforter. It isn't expensive or time-consuming to get. When I need a quick fix, all I need to do is jump in the car and drive to the nearest convenience store. Now I have learned that in order to keep the weight off, I have to find ways to express my feelings. I have to work on feeling safe. Unsafe feelings or vulnerability are major triggers for wanting to eat. John recently told a client in a psychic reading, "Your extra weight is like an umbrella in a rain storm. The umbrella protects you from the rain, just as your weight is protecting you from something. You would not get angry at the umbrella for protecting you from the storm, so don't get angry at the extra weight for protecting you."

If we are to truly manage our weight, it is necessary to honestly look at what purpose it serves. For me, fat is a buffer between myself and the world. It's a way of protecting myself from other people. If I am big, people won't get too close. I am an introvert, a person who needs and likes lots of time alone throughout the day. I need lots of space. The extra weight is my way of making sure that I have enough space to breathe. Being overweight is a great excuse when you don't want to be around a lot of people, for example, "I don't have any clothes that fit, so I might as well stay home."

Extra weight has also served to help me feel more powerful. If I am trying to learn how to share my feelings with others, how to be more spontaneous and less controlled, be heard and understood more by others, it is helpful to feel *big*. If I am physically thin, people won't take me seriously because I look fragile. But if I am physically big, they will see me as a more powerful person and they are likely to take me more seriously. Or so a part of me believes.

Fat has also served to protect me from being attractive or sexual. The main reason I put on weight at age 13 was that it was time to have a boyfriend. Because of all the unresolved issues around sexual abuse and the terror I had with men and boys, weight served as a means of protection. I used every chance I could to bring my weight to their attention. As I stated in Chapter 9, "Pregnancy, Children, and Parenting," there were several reasons why I gained forty pounds during my pregnancy. Food comforted me. I used it as my best friend. Whenever I was depressed, I could reach out for food. The main reason that I allowed myself to put on so much weight was to avoid having to deal with men once I was no longer pregnant. I didn't want to be attractive or sexual again. Being left alone was synonymous with being fat. Thus, fat has long been, and continues to be, a source of protection.

In order to break this cycle of losing and gaining back weight, I have had to look honestly at the pay-offs. This has included learning how to get my needs met without gaining weight. If I need space from people or life, I need to say so, rather than putting on an extra ten or fifteen pounds. If I don't want to be sexual, I need to say no to my partner, rather than trying to make myself unattractive. One of the women in my support group said one day, "How am I going to keep my husband away from me when I lose all this weight?" She went on to say that she hated it when her husband touched her. Rather than confronting the issue directly, she had put on fifty pounds!

I am still in the learning stages of weight control. Learning how to express my feelings. Learning to take care of my needs first. Learning to be more assertive. Learning ways to feel safe without food. Learning ways to get comforted and nurtured without food.

I had a client who came to see me for a weight problem. She was in a twelve-step group for eating disorders but said her weight seemed to be getting worse rather than better. When I asked her if she was in therapy, she said that she didn't think therapy was necessary.

While channeling a healing for her, I looked inside psychically because she had requested a psychic reading along with the physical healing. I saw a little girl running from a woman (her mother) who had tried to strangle her. I saw her father being extremely cruel to her, both verbally and physically.

John told me the only way she felt safe was to get as big as possible so no one would ever hurt her again. She began overeating at age six, shortly after her baby brother was born. She felt she had become invisible to her family because everyone paid attention to the baby rather than to her. She wanted to be bigger so people would notice her, too. Now an adult, she had a serious weight problem. She doesn't trust anyone who tells her they love her. She fears for her life. She resents her brother and all men because they always seem to get more attention than she does. She's afraid of touch. She's extremely sensitive about any criticism, and her way of coping with all of her unresolved issues and pain is to overeat.

Before you check into a weight loss program, take that next diet pill, or buy one more tape about weight loss, do the journal work at the end of this chapter. Your body is suffering from a weight problem for reasons other than you're eating too much. There's much more going on! Be tough with yourself and honestly look at these issues.

If you are overweight, chances are you are very angry with yourself and your body. Remember, the abusive way you talk to yourself will not change your relationship to food or help you lose weight. You are going to have to go within and search out the real issues—what is really eating away at you inside.

Anorexia and Bulimia

Perhaps being overweight is not your food issue. You may be underweight because of anorexia or bulimia. When a person is anorexic, he or she is obsessed with being thin, refusing to eat normally. Bulimics binge on food and then purge themselves so the food cannot fulfill its nutritive role. The use of laxatives, enemas, and suppositories is a sign of bulimic disorders.

I had a client who came in for a psychic reading to help her understand what her anorexia was about. She was in therapy, working hard to recover from anorexia. However, from time to time, she would have a relapse and begin starving herself again. The spirits told her that anorexia is a form of suicide, a sign of resisting change. Her soul, or subconscious, when faced with change and growth from life's lessons, would resist. That resistance would physically manifest itself as starvation.

Another client asked about her bulimia in a psychic reading. The spirits told her that bulimia came from her inner feelings of shame, guilt, and dirtiness as a result of being sexually abused as a child. She was trying to purge herself of these things. She had so much rage and so many frightful feelings that she was continually trying to throw it up or purge it out. This allowed her to avoid having to deal with her real feelings.

Not everyone who has anorexia or bulimia will be exactly like either of the people I describe above. But most of us with a weight issue—whether overweight or underweight—need to understand that it is related to our inner lives. Its roots are emotional. And no diet alone will ever fix that. Exercise isn't the solution either. Compassion, understanding, loving yourself are the ingredients to break the unhealthy weight patterns.

For those of you who aren't certain if you suffer from anorexia or bulimia, here are early symptoms of both, as described by the Golden Valley Health Center (4101 Golden Valley Road, Golden Valley, MN 55422). Also, here is a seven- question quiz to determine if you have an eating problem ranging from bulimia to anorexia.

Eating Disorders

Here are seven statements that can help you determine if you have an eating problem. Check off the ones to which you would answer yes:

1. I often stuff myself with a lot of food in a short period of time.
2. I frequently crave and consume large amounts of junk food or food with high calorie counts.
3. I hide food—or I hide from others while I am eating.
4. I eat until somebody interrupts me, or I feel abdominal pain, or I fall asleep, or I start vomiting.
5. I have tried to lose weight by chronic fasting, severely restricting my diet, by vomiting, by taking laxatives, or by using diuretics.

6. I am afraid that I won't be able to stop myself from eating or I have generally not been able to stop eating voluntarily.
7. I often feel depressed, or guilty, or have harsh thoughts about myself after an eating binge.

This quiz was adapted from questions in the American Psychiatric Association's diagnostic manual.

* * *

If you checked off any of these seven statements, you have an eating problem and should look for medical help, according to Dr. Stanley Title, a prominent New York diet specialist, and Judy Hollis of the Eating Disorders Unit at the CareUnit Hospital of Los Angeles.

If you checked off statements one or two, this indicates an unnatural compulsion to stuff yourself, or a growing addiction to food. Of this Dr. Title warns, "These people overeat because they're seeking emotional comfort from food . . . But people who use food for emotional comfort develop a tolerance and start to need more and more to feel okay," Dr. Title warns.

If you checked off statement three, it indicates that you are aware of a developing abnormal eating problem. People who hide food or hide their eating from others are building a dependency on food that's just like an addict's dependency on drugs, says Hollis.

Anorexia—Early Signs and Symptoms

Check the following statements that you feel apply to you:

1. I will use any means to lose weight.
2. I have the feeling that parts of my body, or even my whole body, is larger than it actually is.
3. I have a frantic preoccupation with food, weight, and sometimes with exercise.
4. I have an intense fear of becoming obese.
5. I impose certain rituals around my food: i.e. cutting up food into minuscule pieces, eating at certain exact hours of the day, etc.
6. I develop sudden and intense interests in books about food, cookbooks, diet books, etc.

7. I have low self-esteem.
8. I am isolated from friends and family.
9. I prefer to eat alone.
10. I have recently experienced sudden weight loss, thinning hair, flaking skin, and loss of menses.
11. I have increased the amount of physical exercise I get.
12. I have difficulty sleeping.
13. I tend to look at things in black and white—all good or all bad, seldom in shades of gray.
14. I have little interest in sex.
15. I experience episodes of fatigue or fainting.
16. I have mood swings.

Bulimia—Early Signs and Symptoms

The following statements are early warning signals of bulimia:

1. I feel very concerned about my weight and will do anything to keep it down.
2. I have a preoccupation with eating and food.
3. I am constantly concerned with my appearance—my feelings of self-worth are based on my weight.
4. I go to the bathroom immediately after meals.
5. I have enlarged parotid glands, giving me a "chipmunk" look.
6. I sometimes find myself sneaking large quantities of food.
7. I am secretive—having difficulty telling the truth to others and sometimes am tempted to steal (or actually do).
8. I isolate myself from friends and family.
9. I have mood swings.
10. I am becoming increasingly impulsive in my behavior.
11. I have difficulty sleeping.

12. I suspect that my use of drugs or alcohol may be getting out of control.
13. I feel tired and apathetic.
14. I suffer from depression.

Whatever behavior patterns you become aware of, remember that you can change them. If you find that you overeat or keep weight on to protect yourself, you can start now to find ways of providing safety for yourself. You can remove yourself from threatening situations. It is important to stay present, focused on the *now,* and praying for the strength you need to get out of any frightening or painful situations. If you feel threatened, call friends and get their support. If you are in a situation where harm can come to you, call 911. Don't hesitate. There are community support groups and other resources to help you with virtually any threatening situation. We can protect ourselves now that we are adults. We do not have to be victims anymore!

Keeping Our Own Counsel

It is difficult to love ourselves when we don't like our physical appearance. But if when you look in the mirror you see a person who is heavier than you want to be, remember that there are reasons for your weight problem. It has literally nothing to do with your lack of will power, so don't wallow in guilt the next time someone tells you that all you need is a little self-control. Remind yourself that it's your body and you don't need other people's judgments.

JOURNAL WORK

In the previous pages, you have read through and perhaps checked off the lists concerning your feelings and behavior around weight. Having done this, and having read this chapter, it can be helpful to record your observations and your discoveries in your journal.

Note things like your relationship with food: What does it do for you? Does it calm you down after a stressful day? Is it your reward for getting through the day? Is it your friend when you are feeling down? When you're feeling lonely? Does it protect you when you feel afraid? Does it distract you from feeling your feelings? Does your weight protect you from getting into a relationship? From being sexual? Do you eat to live or live to eat?

Many experts on weight management say that it is virtually impossible to heal the issues we have around weight without help from at least one other supportive person. That person might be a close friend who is struggling with issues very similar to yours and is also willing to look inside for solutions. Or it might be a therapist, healer, or support group who will provide you with the outside help that will work for you.

The people who are most successful in healing the pain they experience around weight learn all they can about food and eating, perhaps through a weight loss program, and combine this with an in-depth exploration on what purpose food serves in their lives. Keeping a record of your insights, your growing knowledge of food, and its mental and emotional effects on you is an excellent way to keep yourself moving along your own healing path.

The bottom line is:

Our weight issues are no one's business but our own!

We put ourselves through enough shame and guilt around these issues without having to listen to other people's stuff. We have to stop judging ourselves and begin listening to ourselves. Our needs. Our wants. Our fears. Our anxieties. Our *shoulds.*

When the issues underlying our weight are resolved, the fat will literally disappear and, vice-versa, when the issues concerning being underweight get resolved, the weight will stay on and we'll be comfortable with it. Your new body image and perceptions of yourself will manifest themselves. This, coupled with proper exercise and nutrition, will complete your transformation into a place of wellness, safety, and self-respect. You can do it!

CHAPTER 15

Losses and Grieving

Allow yourself your grieving. Allow it to express in whatever way feels right to you. Grieving is the way we heal the loss we feel for someone we love.
—Deborah Duda

Every year between Thanksgiving and Christmas, for as long as I can remember until the age of thirty-five, I would feel a deep sense of loss inside. A deep, deep sadness. It was as though I had lost something really important. No matter how excited I was about the holidays, no matter how busy I was preparing for the holiday season, I would invariably feel a deep gnawing for the entire month. It was as if I had once had something very special and had lost it. Some years I would go into such a deep depression that I would tell my family I just couldn't participate in the holidays. Feeling the heavy sense of loss of something that I didn't even understand, plus baking, shopping, wrapping presents, and tree-trimming, were all just way too much for me.

There was also another feeling that was hard to cope with, a feeling as if I was once special but that something had happened and that specialness had been taken away. Every year I would mentally prepare myself. I would say affirmations, thinking if I was in a good place mentally before December, maybe that would ward off my sadness. Some years I went into therapy, hoping that talking about it in advance would ward it off. No matter what I did, that deep sense of loss would begin all over again.

My wedding date was December 16, 1983. I was sure that when the time approached that year I would be so excited I just wouldn't fall into that all-too-familiar heaviness. But, sure enough, the first week in December rolled around and out came the tears! I always felt so little, as if I was a three-year-old again. I felt vulnerable, afraid, alone, and confused.

What the hell was this all about? Here I was, thirty-five years old, and this damn bogeyman would not go away. I prayed for help. Soon afterwards, I felt intuitively that I should call my mother. At first, my intellect got in the way and said not to bother her with this again, that she'd heard me talk about it for years. We had talked about it so much that there wasn't much more to say. Despite this, I did feel the inner nudging again, so I gave her a call.

Something was different this time. Maybe it was because I finally knew how to express my feelings more clearly or that it was just time for it to be revealed . . . I'm not sure. Maybe it was because this time I said more to my mom than just how sad and empty and depressed I felt, which is what I had always said in the past. Being in therapy was helping me to identify my feelings and talk about them more clearly.

I told my mom that I was feeling that heavy sense of loss again and didn't want it overshadowing the wedding. I just needed to talk through each feeling with her. I needed to tell her it felt as if I was once really special but that this feeling had just vanished from my life. I told her that I felt as if I wanted to go find what I had lost. It felt as if one day, long ago, I had been okay and the next day I was all alone.

As I was sharing these feelings with her, I was sobbing like a baby, which is what I did every December. Feeling the heaviness of my sense of loss and crying. My mom listened carefully to me and suddenly realized what was going on.

She told me that from the time I was a baby until I was four, a person who had dearly loved me was my grandpa. She said he would come over every day to see me. He always read to me, taught me things, and treated me as very special. When I turned three, he discovered he had cancer and so wasn't able to come over every day for our visits. Also, I had a new baby brother. My life was changing.

Mom told me that right after Thanksgiving one year, he got very sick and in December he died. I never saw him after that Thanksgiving. She said they didn't know how to explain death to a four-year-old, so they just never said anything about grandpa. As a little four-year old, all I knew was that my best friend, who had been by my side every day of my life, and who had treated me as very special, never came back. I may have felt that I did something wrong or that his going away had something to do with the new baby. I don't know how I felt or reasoned it out in my childhood mind. We had never talked about my grandfather's death, but all my feelings about that loss were still in there! Every December they reminded me of my loss.

That night and for the next few days, I let myself feel all of it. Whenever my intellect tried to take over and tell me that enough is enough, I told it to stop trying to interfere. I wanted to be free from the sadness. I talked to my grandfather, pretended he was there, and thanked him for all he had given me while he was here. It felt as if a tremendous healing took place over that three-day period. It was wonderful. It's been seven years since that time, and I can honestly say that I have not experienced another black December in all that time.

I can't emphasize enough the importance of getting those feelings of loss out of your body. In my case, those feelings always manifested in my body as digestion problems and headaches throughout the month of December. It was as physically difficult as it was emotionally trying for me during that time of year, until I discovered the truth about the close, loving relationship I had with my grandfather.

Throughout our lives, we suffer from many, many different kinds of losses: the death of a loved one, the break-up of a relationship, the pain of a divorce, or the loss of a home through natural disaster, a fire, or moving to another city. We experience the loss of a job, our health, money, success, a pet, material possessions, teachers, or our youth.

Everyone experiences loss. It's a part of life. When we suffer from a physical injury, we are given time to heal. People send us cards and flowers. Sometimes we are even paid to take time off so we can heal. Unfortunately, when we suffer an emotional injury such as the loss of a loved one, not only are we expected to rise above it and get back to work, oftentimes people don't know what to say to us, so they don't say anything. On top of feeling the loss, we feel terribly alone.

Loss and grief are tough to handle for most of us. Though we lose people and things we hold dear to our hearts throughout our lives, we still don't know what to do with the feelings we have at those times. We don't know how much time we're allowed to grieve the loss. We feel guilty if we don't grieve "appropriately," yet what is appropriate? Most of us don't know what to do. Is it okay to feel pain, cry, yell, scream, be numb, get angry, play sad songs, wallow in memories, and get mad at God? Should we just be inappropriate and really express our total frustration over our powerlessness?

We like to think of ourselves as powerful beings who have control of our lives. But the truth is that, as human beings we are all very vulnerable. Life can change so dramatically for us. It can change with the blink of an eye.

We lose something that is dear to our hearts. We feel devastated, alone, angry, confused, powerless. We want to blame. We run through our list of "if onlys." We do whatever we can to make the pain go away as fast as possible. We search for ways to distract us from our pain. Many of us pretend we're over our pain so that (a) we don't have to feel our feelings; and (b) others don't have to be *bothered* with our feelings, either.

The bottom line is that there is nothing worse than the pain of loss. The bad news is that it hurts like hell and there is no magic pill to relieve it. Even if your doctor gives you a "magic" pill, the pain is still inside and needs to be released. The good news is that time really does heal the pain—if we let it.

Time and *going into* the pain is what brings about the cure. What exactly does this mean? My chiropractor taught me this and it works: When you have a pain, whether it's physical or emotional, take a deep breath and lean into the pain. Don't resist it. The less you resist the pain, the quicker you will come out of it. I'm serious!

Feel the loss. Feel the emptiness. Feel the aloneness. You will not die if you allow yourself to feel it. It will be less stressful on your body if you feel it rather than resist it. Once you allow yourself to go into the pain, your healing process begins. Closing the door on a chapter in our lives is difficult, but not impossible. We do survive loss.

Many ancient teachers have even suggested that there is a positive side of loss and grieving. Black Elk, one of our better known Native American elders, once said that "perhaps the most important reason for 'lamenting' is that it helps us to realize our oneness with all things, to know that all things are our relatives. . . ." (from *Black Elk Speaks*)

Looking At Loss

Our focus in this chapter is to look at losses we have not allowed ourselves to fully experience. Where is our pain sitting? Where in our bodies is it being stored? You may not be able to answer this question right away, and that's okay. It is enough to start this process of letting go by giving some thought to the losses you have had in your life and whether or not you allowed yourself to adequately grieve those losses.

Perhaps you're grieving a loss right now. Do you have any physical pain? The reason I ask about physical pain is that there's a good chance that your body is acting it out in some way, if you're not emotionally grieving the loss. For example, a few years ago my minister died. He had been a mentor of mine for quite awhile. When he was diagnosed with cancer, it was really hard for me to accept. His death shortly thereafter was even harder. I didn't want to feel his loss emotionally.

I was afraid that if I went into the pain of his death, I would be devastated and wouldn't be able to come out of it. On the day of his memorial service, I had the most excruciating lower back pain. I ended up in the emergency room of the hospital. The doctor said there was something wrong with my kidneys, but had no idea what it could be. Kidneys have to do with elimination. I believe that my kidneys were saying to eliminate this pain. Let it out. Stop holding it in. I was fighting the process of grieving my minister's death. I didn't want to go to the memorial service and finally accept his death and my loss. I spent the rest of the day crying about his death. By the end of the day, the lower back pain was gone. These unresolved feelings really do cause us physical pain!

If you discover in doing the journal work at the end of this chapter that you have not grieved over some of your losses, I strongly suggest that you take some time and write out all of your feelings about each loss in your journal. If you feel fearful of becoming overwhelmed with emotion, I recommend that you call a local hospital and see if grief groups are available. If not, ask them whom they would recommend, or ask your doctor or therapist. Grieving does not need to go on forever. When you really face the loss and feel it, when you fully express your feelings about it, you become free to move back into life. By pretending that the feelings of grief are not inside, you become imprisoned by your own feelings. You are not free to live your life spontaneously with an open heart. Pray for the courage to complete your grief and free yourself from the pain of loss. It's worth it!

JOURNAL WORK

Exercise 1

Identifying the Loss

In your journal, make two columns of approximately the same size by drawing a vertical line up the middle of the page. Label the left column "My Losses," the right column, "How I did or didn't respond."

Now, in the corresponding column, write out the losses you have had in your lifetime. Go into as much or as little detail as you wish. Then, in the right column, describe how you responded to that loss. If you felt numb about the loss, or simply didn't respond, write that.

Exercise 2

Losses Experienced From Deep Within

Divide a blank page in your journal with a vertical line up the middle, labeling the left column "Your Child's Losses" and the right column "How You (When a Child) Responded to the Loss."

Put a pencil, pen, or crayon in your nondominant hand and ask your inner child to write about the losses he or she has suffered. Remember, this is a child's response. Their answers will be different than an adult's. The inner child may remember friends, pets, toys, or teachers you have forgotten. The goal here is to get all those losses out of your body and onto paper.

CHAPTER 16

Fear and Resentment

Our society has tremendous prohibitions against feeling too much. We are afraid to feel too much fear, hurt, sadness, or anger; and oftentimes we are also afraid to feel too much love, passion, or joy! And we're definitely afraid of our natural sensuality and sexuality.

—Shakti Gawain

Fear is like an evil ghost. We know that it's there; we pretend it isn't, and we're afraid to do anything about it. So it just takes up residence wherever it feels like and goes on haunting us. But there is good and bad fear and it can be helpful to be able to tell one from the other.

Healthy fear gives us a sense of when something really isn't safe. It warns us of danger. Otherwise, we might all be jumping off cliffs or walking through Central Park alone at night. The good news is that healthy fear isn't going to hurt us. It protects us from getting hurt.

Negative fear, however, can cripple us. It shows up in the body as a very icy-cold energy. Oftentimes, if a person is carrying a great deal of fear, I can feel about five inches of a thick coldness that either sits in certain areas of the body or completely envelops it.

A young woman in her early thirties came to me for a healing that had to do with her fear around love. There were cold spots throughout her body. She had just fallen in love but had many negative messages inside about love: her parents' bitter divorce; disappointing relationships she'd had in the past; painful, past-life memories concerning love, of which she wasn't conscious but were there nonetheless. She really felt her new love was right for her in many ways, and she did not want anything to interfere with the potential she believed this relationship had. Yet, the fear was holding her back. She discovered that she was going to be able to go forward and let that relationship unfold only if she learned to release herself from the negative images of the past that she was still holding in her body.

Fear and Physical Pain

A few years ago I was in the hospital, waiting to undergo my fourth surgery in two years. It was to be the second surgery on my colon. I was very upset that I was back in the hospital and that I was still in pain after three other attempts to correct the problem. Why was I going through all of this? Was it some karmic debt from another lifetime being manifested? I felt very frustrated that I couldn't see for myself what was going on. Here I was, a psychic who had helped many other people understand why they went through similar situations, yet I couldn't see what was going on with me!

My mom called a Medicine Man she knew in South Dakota and asked him if he could see why I was back in this same predicament. He called me at the hospital the day before the surgery to tell me he'd had a vision of my colon and that it was full of fear. I had stored all my fear and fearful memories inside since childhood. He said that I had to work on releasing all the fears that I stored in my colon if I ever wanted it to work properly.

When I hung up the phone, I felt overwhelmed. Where in the world was I going to begin? I had hoped that he would give me some magical words; then I could pack my bags and go home. The last thing I wanted to hear was that I had to eliminate all the fear from my lifetime that I was storing in my colon. I felt so alone and so afraid. There was a part of me that knew he was right, even though intellectually I wasn't yet convinced that stored emotions could have such a devastating effect on my body.

I had the surgery. The doctor corrected the physical problem by removing thirteen inches of twisted intestines. I knew intuitively that I needed to work on surrendering my fears rather than holding onto them. I did not want to have any more surgery or any more pain. I wanted to heal.

It took time for me to be honest with myself. I remembered my first reaction when the Medicine Man told me the problem was fear: "No way do I have any fear. I am tough. I can handle anything." The truth was that I was very fearful despite the fact that I was handling things. It took me a long time to be willing to see it.

I believe that all of us who are traveling a spiritual path eventually need to face our fears. We can't in all honesty say that we're faith-filled, if in fact we are fear-filled. If there is an inner conflict between faith and fear, we must work on resolving it. Emmanuel says, "People have to deal with fear because it is one of the greatest denials of the reality of God." (*Emmanuel's Book,* p. 164)

It's taken me awhile, but I think that I have identified most of my fears. I find now when I get a pain in my colon that I am going through something in my life that's causing me to feel afraid. It's time for me to surrender those fears once again. See the list on page 135 of the fears that I came up with. As you're reading my list, I would like you to start becoming aware of what your fears may be, so you can make up your own and record it in your journal.

Resentments

Resentments, like fear, have the ability to make our life miserable. Fortunately, both are totally under our control. What is a resentment? Webster's dictionary defines resentment as taking "strong exception to what is thought to be unjust, interfering, insulting, critical, etc." To me, it's remembering a hurt that has been done to me and not wanting to let it go—harboring angry or hateful feelings. By holding onto resentments, we can think of many ways to get back at the person who hurt us: revenge, plotting, obsessions, etc. It can get quite serious if we hold onto the injuries other people have inflicted upon us; these seemingly harmless little feelings can cause serious damage in our bodies.

As a healer, I have seen that resentments can be the root cause of physical problems. When you have resentment towards someone, where do you think it is stored? It stays stored somewhere in your body. Yes, it does! Resentments don't just reside somewhere in your mental memory bank. They will find a comfortable place somewhere in your body and rest there until you do something with them—and this means either getting back at the person or letting the resentment go. If you make a statement to yourself such as, "I will never forget what so-and-so did to me," you are consciously storing that memory

My List of Fears

Fear of being alone

Fear of not being wanted

Fear of not being special enough to someone

Fear of not being needed

Fear of not being loved

Fear of not being accepted

Fear of not being cool

Fear of losing different people who have been in my life

Fear of illness

Fear of separation from my family

Fear of being physically abused

Fear of being sexually abused

Fear of dying

Fear of living

Fear of doctors

Fear of the dentist

Fear of taxes/the IRS

Fear of my business failing

Fear of becoming crippled

Fear of burning in a fire

Fear of losing my sight

Fear of breaking a bone

Fear of succeeding

Fear of others competing with me

Fear of being a wash-out in sports or general activities

Fear of criticism

Fear of "doing it wrong"

Fear of getting pregnant

Fear of not getting pregnant

Fear of being a wimp

Fear of my feelings

Fear of people I love dying

Fear of being poor

Fear of God not really being there

Fear of responsibility

Fear of recognition

Fear of non-recognition

Fear of more physical pain

Fear of never being understood by anyone

Fear of driving on the freeway

Fear of drowning

Fear of mice

Fear of something bad happening to my niece and nephew

Fear of my sister getting sick again

Fear of losing my house

Fear of letting a client down

Fear that no one will read my books

Fear (when I was married) that my husband would have affairs

Fears that my marriage would not work

in your body, along with the bitterness and hatred. Our resentments become bitter stories that grow with the passing of time.

The story of a client whose hearing was bad in one ear comes to mind. His story, which he told every time he came in for a healing, was that he had been hunting with his best friend. His friend shot at a duck just as my client was moving towards him. The gun went off right in his ear. The first time that he told me the story, the mishap seemed quite unintentional. But I found that each time he told me the story, depending on what kind of a day he was having, the story would change. Once, when he came for his appointment, he was in a bad mood; nothing had gone right for him at work and his kids were bugging him. When he told me the story of losing his hearing, he said his friend tried to kill him! I suggested to him that he needed to think about forgiving his friend and letting the story go so his ear would have a chance to heal.

Your body will store your story somewhere so you can always dredge up the facts and tell it over and over again. Somehow, we think that if we never forgive and forget the people who hurt us, that they will suffer the punishment. The simple truth is that we're the ones who end up crippled with arthritis, back pain, headaches, cancer, or whatever. The resentment is killing us, not the people we find it so hard to forgive.

Many people don't know any other way to get attention or sympathy or love than to share their stories about how they've been hurt. They tell their stories over and over again, telling anyone and everyone who'll listen all the details about "who done them wrong."

Every day, people intentionally or unintentionally hurt us. Most often it's unintentional. Each time a hurt comes our way, we have the choice to either let it go or hang onto it and store it away until we can get back at them. We believe we will be able to rest only when we feel that justice has been served. But as quickly as justice is served in one case, another injustice is there to take its place, because the act of resenting has become a habit. From a physical standpoint, this can be very harmful. I have seen clients terribly crippled from past resentments.

One characteristic of resentment is that it is often not as obvious to us as it is to others. As an example, a woman came to me for healings on a sprained ankle. Her story was that a male friend had been staying with her and one day, in a big hurry, needed her to drive him somewhere. In the pressure of hurrying, she tripped and fell, spraining her ankle. The man never offered to help her, nor did he apologize for making her rush. He just continued to be in a hurry, thus making her feel as if she was a klutz.

It took months for this woman's sprained ankle to heal. The healing was finally complete when she let go of her resentment, which she was holding onto as a desire to have him acknowledge her difficulty. It was only through a psychic reading that we learned that she was subconsciously holding onto this resentment. As soon as she became conscious of her resentment, and her desire for his acknowledgment, she was able to let it go. The pain in her ankle quickly went away after thereafter.

Often when people are waiting for someone to apologize to them (or at least acknowledge the misdeed in some way) and the person responds in some positive manner, the healing takes place almost instantaneously. Likewise, when we forgive the person whom we believe caused our problem, the same thing will happen—even though the other person doesn't do what we desire. Unfortunately, most people don't openly acknowledge their part in hurting us. That's why it's up to the person who's been hurt to let go of the resentment and stop waiting for the other person to make it all right. Forgiveness is a choice we make to let go of those harsh feelings we are holding inside, not necessarily because we want to let the other person off the hook but because we no longer want these feelings to hurt us. Above all, it is a choice for health.

If you can still remember something that happened to you a long time ago, and you still have feelings about it, it is still being held inside of you and is a potential danger to your health! Don't minimize these nasty critters. Here is a short list of people and institutions that may have caused you harm in some way in the past. Use the list to jar your memory loose of any old, forgotten resentments: Parents, sisters and brothers, grandparents, uncles, aunts, cousins, nieces, nephews, babysitters, teachers, ministers, priests, rabbis, doctors, dentists, friends, bosses, co-workers, children, neighbors, animals, police, city governments, building inspectors, insurance companies, automobile manufacturers, hospitals, prisons, nursing homes, welfare systems, educational systems, the Veterans Administration, the Department of Natural Resources, and the Internal Revenue Service.

When We Have Hurt Others

Another area of the resentment issue that is not so pleasant to look at has to do with the pain we have caused others. The eighth step of AA's twelve-step program is: "Made a list of all persons we have harmed and became willing to make amends to them all." Step nine is: "Made direct amends to such people wherever possible, except when to do so would injure them or others."

Apropos of this, in a movie called *Flatliners* five young doctors assist each other in near-death experiences. Instead of the white light of heaven, however, three of them are haunted by memories of people they harmed in their lives. Another doctor experiences all of her repressed guilt from feeling responsible for her father's death. One of the doctors suggests that they make amends to these people whom they have hurt. He himself does this and finds peace of mind. The experiences dramatized in this movie are not unlike experiences that many people have in real life, where they encounter death or a serious illness, and suddenly see how their own healing is related to processes such as forgiveness or making amends.

What are amends? Webster says: "To correct, to improve; to change or revise." It's not only apologizing for the hurt that we have caused others, it's changing our future behavior toward that person. The apology isn't much good if we apologize for something and then turn right around and do it again! What is most important of all is changing our own behavior.

I know that making a list of people you have harmed is not a pleasant thought, but it's necessary to your healing. Sometimes people get stuck in saying: "Well, so and so hurt me more. So I don't need to make amends to them." Don't get stuck there! This taking care of your unfinished business is *for your sake, your healing*. It has nothing to do with our everyday concepts of justice.

It can be helpful to ask God, the Universe, or whatever is your concept of a *higher power* to help you be willing to list those hurts that you have caused others. Slowly, you will discover in yourself the desire to look at this. When this desire does come, record your findings in your journal.

As you are making amends, look at the possibility of forgiving people who have caused you harm. This is the other side of making amends, with the act of forgiveness freeing us from past hurts. It's a tough one, I know! Forgive others and let it go. Let go of the person, the circumstances, and the stories.

In making amends to people you have harmed, be very careful not to injure anybody in the process. Let me explain. In many cases, we may feel we have done harm but if we think about how we are going to make amends, we may discover that some part of doing so might actually cause injury to another person.

When considering making amends, ask yourself if the amendment you are thinking about is going to make the other person feel better. If it may cause the other more harm, don't do it. While the purpose of making amends is to clean out all the old guilt and shame, as well as to wipe the slate clean, it is not to be done at another's expense! In many cases, the very best way we can make amends is to forgive ourselves for the harm we caused.

Both of these lists—resentments we have as well as the harm we have caused others—will stay with you until you take care of the business by forgiving them, letting them go, and making amends.

So why not just take care of all of both complete and total lists right now? The main reason is that something like this takes time. To have the lists available to us in our journal gives us a way to keep in mind what we have to do.

You can't imagine how freeing these processes can be! You know how good it feels to clean out closets and drawers and get rid of things you no longer need or want. That's how forgiving, letting go, and making amends can feel! You'll feel as if fifty pounds has been lifted from you.

If you're not sure about forgiveness and letting go, read the "Forgiveness" chapter in Section II, Solutions, on page 211. It really is helpful. Do this for your sake. You don't need to keep carrying all this old stuff with you.

JOURNAL WORK

FEARS

Exercise 1
Listing Your Fears

In your journal, make a list of your fears. Remember that you are doing this just for you. List every fear that comes into your mind, no matter how petty it may seem. List them even though you may think they are "silly" or unjustified. In making my own list, I found that some of them were embarrassing to admit. But if this bothers you, remember that you don't have to share this list with anyone. The purpose here is to start getting these fears out of your body and down on paper where they can do you no harm.

Exercise 2
Feeling Your Fear

When you've finished your list, sit down and feel your body. Are you aware of pain anywhere? Did you have pain in any part of your body while you were making this list? Jot it down here. Make a list of the physical pains you associate with each of your fears.

Exercise 3
The Inner Child

Part A

With your nondominant hand, ask your inner child to share with you what fears he or she has. Remember, your inner child's list may be very different from your adult's list. Be patient. She or he may be afraid to tell you about these fears, so I would encourage you to remind your inner child that she or he is safe, that you will protect him or her. You may need to ask your inner child two or three times what these fears are.

Have your inner child simply make a list of these fears.

Part B

After your inner child has finished listing her fears, ask what you can do now to help her feel less fearful. Ask her what she needs from you so that she doesn't experience her fear any more. Assure her that you would be willing to do what it is she needs. Remember, her fears are just as real and important as yours. Her fears are controlling your life. It is time to heal.

Have your inner child list what she needs from you to feel safe.

RESENTMENTS

Exercise 4

Listing Resentments

Part A

Divide one or more pages in your journal into three columns. Label the first one, "Name of Person/Organization;" label the middle one, "What They Did to Me;" label the third one, "My Feelings Then and Now."

Now get mentally in touch with people, organizations, and institutions toward whom you feel resentment. Write down the name, then tell what they did to you. Lastly, record your feelings around that event—both what you felt when it first happened and what you are feeling now.

Part B

The founders of Alcoholics Anonymous believed that to stop drinking permanently, alcoholics had to let go of past resentments. I believe that our resentments hinder any healing process tremendously.

When you're done listing the resentments you're aware of, go to a close friend or relative and ask them if you have any resentments that they're aware of. Often, we are not aware of our own stories. We may not even be aware of all the war stories we tell but our close friends may be able to tell us word for word what they are. If after talking with a friend you discover more resentments that you have, add them to your list.

Exercise 5
Making Amends

Divide one or more journal pages into three columns again, this time labeling them, respectively: "People I Have Harmed," "What I Did to Them," and "How I Will Make Amends."

Now fill in the blank spaces. Remember the cautions about making amends only if they will do no harm. And remember, too, that sometimes the most healing way you can make amends is to find it in your heart to forgive yourself.

CHAPTER 17

Stress and Depression

Your symptoms may not be in your head, but the power to get rid of them may well be.
—STUART BERGER, M.D.

Sometimes stress and depression go together like a hand in a glove. But not always. So we'll address them separately in this chapter.

What is stress? Stress is your body's reaction to any conflicting or excessive demands placed upon it. Have you ever gone to your doctor with some physical problem, only to have him or her say: "I can't find anything wrong. It must be stress"? It's interesting to me that the statement, "it must be stress," somehow minimizes the physical or emotional problem that person is having. There's also an unspoken message there that implies that we should just "cope better" with our lives.

Do you ever stop and think how much you go through each day? Each day we perform our routines, interact with other people, and make decisions for our lives and others. We eat food to maintain our bodies. Usually we get a minimal amount of exercise. We sleep five to nine hours per night. We work eight to ten hours per day. We pay the bills. We earn more money so we can pay more bills.

Challenges face us at every turn. Our minds are constantly engaged, both in thinking through the moment or racing ahead to plan for what must be done next. Our feelings are always operating at some level, whether or not we are aware of them. While we may be feeling that we are alone on our journey through life, it is seldom that we are truly alone. There is always someone to focus our attention on: children, parents, other family members, and friends.

Add to this scenario additional factors such as: bill collectors, health emergencies, deaths, accidents, holidays, unexpected work or school assignments, traffic delays, schedules running behind due to circumstances beyond our control, phone lines busy, computers shutting down, threatening mail, the school nurse calling to say that your child needs to come home, long lines at the check-out counter, a flat tire or other car trouble, the bus breaking down, changes in the company management, appointments getting canceled or changed. Any one of us could go on and on with all the unexpected stresses that can come up in the course of any day.

Think for a moment about how much you go through each day: mentally, emotionally, physically, and spiritually. Trace the events of a typical day. Most of us do not realize how much stress we place on our bodies and minds. We take life's demands with a grain of salt and scarcely even notice our daily challenges until we become completely exhausted or ill.

The only way for our body to get our attention when it is feeling burned out or stressed to the limit is to send some kind of signal that something is wrong. I took a stress management class to learn how to cope with stress. In the class, we listed the physical symptoms people experience as a result of stress. Here is a list of the health problems we came up with:

aches	diarrhea
hyperventilation	alcohol abuse
disassociation	impotence
anxiety attacks	drug abuse
insomnia	back pains
eating disorders	jaw tightness
bladder problems	eye strain
cancer	manic-depressive syndrome
over-stimulation	canker sores
headaches	paranoia
fatigue	colitis
heart attacks	prostate problems
constipation	hemorrhoids
smoking	death
herpes	stroke
diabetes	hypertension
sexual dysfunction	vaginal infection

Rating Your Burn-out Level

Often, we don't even recognize the early signs of burn-out when they occur. When we're in the middle of it, we're too depleted to see what's happening to us. The following test was derived from the work of Dr. Herbert J. Freudenberger, author of a book entitled *Burn Out*:

The Test

Start by looking back over the past six months. Mentally note if there have been any changes at the office, with the family, in your social situations. Have you noticed any changes in yourself or in the way you have been relating to the world around you? Give yourself about thirty seconds to think about each of the following fifteen questions. Then rate yourself on each point according to a scale of 1 to 5, with 5 meaning that you've experienced the most change, 1 being the least.

1. Have you noticed that you tire more easily lately? Do you generally feel fatigued rather than energetic?
2. Have people begun telling you that you don't look so good lately?
3. Does it seem that you are working harder and accomplishing less and less?
4. Are you increasingly cynical or disenchanted?
5. Do you experience sudden spells of sadness you can't explain?
6. Are you becoming forgetful about appointments and deadlines, or are you losing the car keys or misplacing personal objects?
7. Are you becoming increasingly irritable or short-tempered? Or are you feeling more disappointed than usual in the people around you?
8. Are you visiting with close friends and family members less often?
9. Are you so busy that you can't find the time to do routine things such as making phone calls, reading reports, or sending out your Christmas cards?
10. Do you have nagging physical complaints such as aches and pains, headaches, a lingering cold or sinus infection?

11. Do you feel disoriented at the end of the day when you have completed your usual activities?
12. Are you missing any sense of joy in your life?
13. Have you lost your sense of humor about yourself?
14. Has sexual activity become more trouble than it's worth?
15. Do you feel you have very little to say to people?

Tally up your total points and roughly rate yourself on the burn-out scale below. Keep in mind that this is only a rough approximation, useful as a guide for reducing stress in your life. Don't be alarmed if you get a high stress rating. But don't ignore it, either. Burn-out is reversible, no matter how far along it is. But higher ratings suggest that the sooner you start being kinder to yourself, the better.

The Burn-Out Scale

0–25	Okay. You are handling stress well.
26–35	Pay attention. There are areas of stress you should be reducing or eliminating.
36–50	Caution. You could be a candidate for burn-out.
51–65	Trouble. You are burning out.
Over 65	Danger! You are definitely in a dangerous place, one that could threaten your physical and mental well-being.

One area in our lives that I see causing a tremendous amount of stress, anxiety, and worry is money. What a curse that stuff can be! If we don't have enough, we're stressed. If we have a lot, we're stressed in a different way.

It is so important to find a way to express the pressures and stresses we feel in our lives. Talk about them, whatever they may be. Do you have someone in your family or a close friend who is seriously ill or perhaps even dying? That is a major stress for everyone concerned. Have you got troubles on the job? Problems in a relationship? With your children? Health issues yourself? Roommate problems? How about your finances? Maybe you've got a new baby in the house, or a new pet? Even those situations that bring joy can cause extra stress. We all tend to minimize stress, and it's time to stop doing that! We need to acknowledge its impact on us, mentally and physically. Don't just tell yourself you've got to learn how to *cope* better.

In AA, the tenth step states that we "continued to take personal inventory, and when we were wrong, promptly admitted it." What this step suggests is that part of our healing process is to take stock of all the events that took place during the day and look carefully at our reaction(s) to them. If we got uptight with a client or customer, for example, and yelled at them, take note of that. Acknowledge what we did and without judging whether it was right or wrong, simply look at the results. Did it bring greater peace of mind or less? By noting our reactions to stress in this way, we can become more aware of what we do to express or not express it, and that opens up the possibility of changing those patterns. As our awareness increases, we may be encouraged to seek ways to minimize our reaction to stress so that we don't become overwhelmed or ill. The tenth step also suggests righting any wrongs we have done to others during the day as soon as possible.

All twelve-step groups strongly suggest living your life one day at a time, because realistically, that's all we've got. It's much easier to cope with life when we deal with life this way. Finishing up business is what I think of when I read the tenth step. I think this is a wonderful way to minimize the stress from spilling over from one day into the next.

I would like to suggest that from now on, at the end of each day, you take five minutes and review what has occurred. Are you still holding stress from the day's events in your body? Exactly what happened to cause you to feel stressful? Write it down in your journal. What we want to do here is eliminate it at the end of the day, so when you wake up the next morning, you have a fresh start.

Don't underestimate the effects that stress can have on you. It's not worth it to pretend that you can handle it. Yes, we can handle a lot of stress, but why should we have to? We can often get rid of stress by writing it down or talking it out with another person. Another discipline that helps us minimize the effects of stress is learning to live a day at a time. It sounds so simple, but realistically, it's tough! We all want to jump ahead; we want to anticipate, to know what's coming. We want to plan. We want to be ready. We hate not being in control. Try it anyway. Life will become much easier, I promise you!

Depression

Up until seven years ago, I suffered from a manic-depressive disorder. That's what the psychological tests have always called it. I would have extreme mood swings. When I was manic, I would feel on top of the world. I would talk a lot. I'd feel like shouting or screaming in delight, but there wasn't anything to shout or scream about. You know that feeling when you're small and waiting for Santa Claus or your birthday party or a trip to your favorite amusement park? You feel like you're going to jump out of your skin, you're so excited.

That's what the manic side of my cycle felt like, but it's more intense. You literally feel like the top of your head is going to fly off with excitement. The good news is that it doesn't last long. The bad news is that you come down. Way down. You crash into the depression part of manic depression. There is nothing in my life that I ever dreaded more than the onset of depression.

For all of you who do suffer from depression, who have possibly even considered suicide, I hope you will hear these words. Depression is treatable! You don't have to be a victim of this for the rest of your life!

Today as I was trying to prepare myself mentally to write about my old nemesis, I was reading through *Depression and Its Treatment* by John H. Griest, M.D. and James W. Jefferson, M.D. I wanted to refresh my memory of the pain that I once thought I would never be able to forget. In the chapter on "What Is Depression," they include a patient's story describing her depression. As I was reading her story, flashes of old memories came to me. Old pain, frustration, loneliness. That incredible despair that no one seems to understand unless they have been there. The helplessness. The hopelessness and emptiness. The aloneness of not being able to describe that inner desperation. The past, present, and future all feel heavy, bleak, and useless.

Reading the story made me feel very afraid. I didn't want to write about depression. I wanted to forget about it and go on to something else. I felt really anxious inside. I began to fear that if I sat here thinking about it too much, it would find me again after these many years free of it. I got out my vacuum cleaner and furiously vacuumed my house. I didn't feel much relief. I decided to mow my grass. I was observing myself go through all of this. One part of me was saying, "Are you crazy? It's ninety degrees outside and you have to get this chapter written!" But there was another part of me that had to get away from my desk and do something physical. I mowed my lawn as if someone were chasing me. I had headphones on with the music blasting. Memories flooded my mind of past depressions. I felt anger about having gone through all of them. I felt sorry for myself. I remembered all the times I'd tried to explain to people how I felt and realized how futile it was to even try. This always made me feel crazier and more alone than ever. Each time a bout would come, I weighed the pros and cons of suicide. I was always wondering why this was happening to me. Nothing specific seemed to trigger the onset of a depression. Yet slowly it would creep in, and then after a time, sometimes after days, weeks, or months, it would just stop.

Three out of six members of my family suffer from depression. My therapist said it was no wonder I married a man who also suffered from depression. Once when my ex-husband and I were in counseling, our therapist told him he needed to deal with his depression before any other changes could occur in his life or in our marriage. He fought accepting his depression, just as I did when I was diagnosed as a manic-depressive. We both hated the label. My ex-husband eventually tried medication for his depression and it made a tremendous difference for him. Mine stopped when I really started looking at all of my issues that I have talked about in this book.

Today, I believe that all the pain and memories, unresolved issues, feelings, and beliefs sitting inside would just throw my body into overwhelm. Then, in a sense, I would break down and get depressed. Different therapists suggested various medications over the years, but because of my former addiction to pills, I was very leery of taking anything. My AA sponsor worked with me on the depression. He, too, had suffered from manic-depressive disorder. When I would begin going into the manic high, he would tell me over and over, "Bring those highs down and those lows up. Don't let yourself go so high or get so low." It did help, even though it was difficult to do because when someone is depressed, they don't care. It was tough to fight that apathy.

First let me tell you the woman's story that appeared in the book on the treatment of depression which I read that day. See if it sounds like anything you are going through.

Prior to the onset of her depression, the woman said she felt elated because she had given birth to twins two months earlier. At first she tried to keep her mind occupied by doing busy-work around the house—cleaning, watching after the babies, etc. However, she found she had no enthusiasm for anything she was doing. She was getting no pleasure at all from living. She felt nothing toward her babies or her other two children. She tried to do extra things for the children because she felt so guilty about not loving them. She would do everything in the house quickly and then would find herself with nothing to do. She had no interest in outside activities or projects which would be of great interest to her when she wasn't feeling depressed. She found she couldn't concentrate on anything. Her mind seemed to dwell exclusively on black thoughts. Her husband took her out frequently, trying to get her to take her mind off things, but even that was a tremendous effort for her and she seldom got much enjoyment from it.

Time passed and this woman's feelings of despair and hopelessness got worse. She lost weight and had no appetite. She would try to sleep away her days but this didn't work. She had terrible dreams and would often wake up in a panic. Feelings of anxiety were always present. For no reason that she could explain, her symptoms continued to worsen. She found herself not wanting to go home when she went out shopping, yet she couldn't stand to be alone. No matter what she did, she couldn't concentrate on any thoughts except her own self-doubts about her sanity or why she deserved what she was feeling.

She felt that her appearance had changed radically. She felt old and ugly. She had no sexual desire and was becoming more and more guilty about her lack of desire for any kind of intimacy with her husband. She wondered if she was ever going to get through menopause.

She began going to sleep earlier at night and sleeping as late as possible in the morning. This was the only way she could stop from thinking the same anxious thoughts over and over again. She began to feel physically ill, her appetite dwindled, and she started smoking more. Her stomach began to trouble her, and she developed severe daily headaches. One morning she just couldn't get out of bed. Because she felt physically ill and was unable to take care of her family she began to think that she had a virus and asked her husband to contact the family doctor. The doctor gave her a thorough physical exam with blood tests and urinalysis, but found absolutely nothing wrong. The woman persuaded the doctor to treat her for a possible infection anyway. He didn't tell her that her symptoms could be depression.

Several days later, after taking medication, she felt no improvement. In fact, she woke up one morning and felt she didn't want to live any longer. Nothing in life seemed important or worthwhile, and she began thinking about ways to commit suicide. Her own thoughts racked her entire body with fear. She knew then that she was not physically sick and that she had to reach out for another kind of help. She told this to her husband and saw her physician again. Upon hearing what she had to say, the doctor prescribed an anti-depressant and a tranquilizer. He didn't seem to know much about depression or what kind of medication might help. He recommended that she see a psychiatrist, which she decided she couldn't possibly do. After taking the medications for one day she was even worse. It was her belief that if she needed to see a psychiatrist, it probably meant she was losing her mind, and this thought frightened her even more. She couldn't stand it any longer. The fear of being mentally ill was so horrible that she decided to take the entire bottle of sleeping pills the doctor had prescribed.

While the woman did not succeed in her suicide attempt, she might well have done so had her physician not followed up by referring her to a psychiatrist. She eventually went on a course of medication that relieved her symptoms, allowing her to feel hopeful again. With a follow-up program involving verbal therapy and feeling her feelings, she fully recovered and today is living a normal life.

If you suspect that you suffer from depression, whether it's every day or only periodically, I suggest that you answer the questions in the following questionnaire.

Beck Depression Inventory (BDI)

"This questionnaire contains groups of statements. Please read each group of statements carefully. Then pick out the one statement in each group which best describes the way you have been feeling the *past week, including today.* Circle the number beside the statement you picked. If several statements in the group seem to apply equally, circle the highest number. Be sure to read all the statements in each group before making your choice.

1.0 I do not feel sad.
1 I feel sad.
2 I am sad all the time and I can't snap out of it.
3 I am so sad or unhappy that I can't stand it.

2.0 I am not particularly discouraged about the future.
1 I feel discouraged about the future.
2 I feel I have nothing to look forward to.
3 I feel that the future is hopeless and that things cannot improve.

3.0 I do not feel like a failure.
1 I feel I have failed more than the average person.
2 As I look back on my life, all I can see is a lot of failures.
3 I feel I am a complete failure as a person.

4.0 I get as much satisfaction out of things as I used to.
1 I don't enjoy things the way I used to.
2 I don't get real satisfaction out of anything anymore.
3 I am dissatisfied or bored with everything.

5.0 I don't feel particularly guilty.
1 I feel guilty a good part of the time.
2 I feel quite guilty most of the time.
3 I feel guilty all the time.

6.0 I don't feel I am being punished.
1 I feel I may be punished.
2 I expect to be punished.
3 I feel I am being punished.

7.0 I don't feel disappointed in myself.
1 I am disappointed in myself.
2 I am disgusted with myself.
3 I hate myself.

8.0 I don't feel I am any worse than anybody else.
1 I am critical of myself for my weaknesses or mistakes.
2 I blame myself all the time for my faults.
3 I blame myself for everything bad that happens.

9.0 I don't have any thoughts of killing myself.
1 I have thoughts of killing myself, but I would not carry them out.
2 I would like to kill myself.
3 I would kill myself if I had the chance.

10.0 I don't cry any more than usual.
1 I cry more now than I used to.
2 I cry all the time now.
3 I used to be able to cry, but now I can't cry even though I want to.

11.0 I am no more irritated now than I ever am.
1 I get annoyed or irritated more easily than I used to.
2 I feel irritated all the time now.
3 I don't get irritated at all by the things that used to irritate me.

12.0 I have not lost interest in other people.
1 I am less interested in other people than I used to be.
2 I have lost most of my interest in other people.
3 I have lost all of my interest in other people.

13.0 I make decisions as well as I ever could.
1 I put off making decisions more than I used to.
2 I have greater difficulty in making decisions than before.
3 I can't make decisions at all anymore.

14.0 I don't feel I look any worse than I used to.
1 I am worried that I am looking old or unattractive.
2 I feel that there are permanent changes in my appearance that make me look unattractive.
3 I believe that I look ugly.

15.0 I can work about as well as before.
1 It takes extra effort to get started doing something.
2 I have to push myself very hard to do anything.
3 I can't do any work at all.

16.0 I can sleep as well as usual.
1 I don't sleep as well as I used to.
2 I wake up 2–3 hours earlier than usual and find it hard to get back to sleep.
3 I wake up several hours earlier than I used to and cannot get back to sleep.

17.0 I don't get more tired than usual.
1 I get tired more easily than I used to.
2 I get tired from doing almost anything.
3 I am too tired to do anything.

18.0 My appetite is no worse than usual.
1 My appetite is not as good as it used to be.
2 My appetite is muh worse now.
3 I have no appetite at all anymore.

19.0 I haven't lost much weight, if any, lately.
1 I have lost more than 5 pounds.
2 I have lost more than 10 pounds.
3 I have lost more than 15 pounds.

20.0 I am no more worried about my health than usual.
1 I am worried about physical problems such as aches and pains;or upset stomach; or constipation.
2 I am very worried about physical problems and it's hard to think about anything else.
3 I am so worried about my physical problems that I cannot think about anything else.

21.0 I have not noticed any recent change in my interest in sex.
1 I am less interested in sex than I used to be.
2 I am much less interested in sex now.
3 I have lost interest in sex completely.

"The BDI is scored by adding the numbers of the separate items selected. Do not score weight lost on purpose (item 19). A score of 0–9 would be considered in the normal range, 10–15 would suggest mild depression, 16–23 would be consistent with moderate depression, and a score of 24 or more suggests marked depression.

"We feel anyone who scores between 10 and 23 should repeat the BDI in two weeks. If the score is still between 10 and 23, and particularly if it has risen, a doctor should be consulted for an evaluation. If the score is greater than 23, a prompt evaluation is certainly indicated. If the score is less that 10 but other indications of depression exist, evaluation is also wise." (The BDI and scoring instruction are reprinted from John W. Griest and James W. Jefferson's book, *Depression and Its Treatment,* pp. 22-26, by permission of the publisher, American Psychiatric Press, Inc., Washington, D.C., published in 1985.)

* * *

If you find you do suffer from depression, seek professional help. Don't try to fix it on your own. If you could, you would have done so by now! You're not an expert. Even if you are an expert and are suffering from it, get some help! *You do not have to live with depression.*

You won't necessarily be put on drugs, but if so, there are many new drugs that don't have all of the side effects old medications had. In fact, most people who have serious chronic depression are able to work with a psychiatrist to get exactly the right medication, one that will have few or no side-effects whatsoever. You may have a chemical imbalance in your body. You should not be the judge of what's right for you until you talk to a professional and find out what your options are.

For those of you who are contemplating suicide, you're not going to like it when I tell you this . . . but as a psychic, I have seen souls who have taken their lives because of depression. You are not free from depression just because you leave your physical body. That depression is deep in your soul. It needs to heal, but death will not heal it. The depression will follow you wherever you are. Death is not the answer to depression. It is a problem with known solutions that are sometimes surprisingly simple. If you have a therapist or a doctor who does not take you seriously, who is not helping you to find solutions, find yourself a new one.

If you are not getting what you need to change your depressed state (and I'm not talking about getting stoned on tranquilizers to numb you out) or you don't have a competent doctor who understands how to treat depression (psychiatrists, who are also M.D.s, are trained in this) and a competent therapist who believes that your past affects your future, who encourages you to look at all the unresolved pain inside, switch to another doctor and therapist now. Thousands of people are successfully treated for depression every day.

I am currently working with a client who comes every week for healings for her depression. I lay my hands on her, channeling a healing to release whatever issues are inside her body. Each week a different issue comes up: painful memories of her mother; hurt and disappointment in her marital relationship; negative beliefs that say she's unlovable, unworthy, bad, a burden, incapable, inferior, inadequate, unwanted, worthless. She is seeing me, a therapist, and a chiropractor. She has suffered from depression most of her life and finally got tired of it, deciding that instead of being a victim, she'd do whatever she could to heal it. She is making daily progress in her healing, taking charge of her life, and no longer allowing depression to stop her from going forward.

In a psychic reading, John gave her this prayer to say each day to help with the healing:

> *Don't let me stay stuck in my negativity, in my anger. Push me past the place I am now. Push me. Push me to go deeper in my relationship with God and myself. Push me. Help me change my patterns . . . to see myself as a different person . . . a child of God who is capable of anything. Help me take the blinders off my eyes and see myself clearly. Thank you.*

If you are feeling stuck, I suggest that you say this every day for thirty days. Watch yourself begin to move past the pain of depression. Remember what I said in the beginning of this chapter: I had to read a book to remind myself of the pain of depression. Hopefully, you will be able to say that same thing some day, making your depression a thing of the past.

Are Holidays Depressing?

Holidays can be wonderful, bringing family and friends together. People express love and joy for each other. But holidays can also be awful. They can remind us of the unhealed separation and hurt in our lives.

Holidays are filled with feelings. For instance, there are usually two very distinct reactions to Christmas: People are either totally into it or they hate it. Some people don't react to it one way or another. The same is true to a lesser or greater degree with all the holidays: Hanukkah, Thanksgiving, New Year's Eve, Valentine's Day, Easter, as well as the one special day that is not considered a legal holiday but is, I believe a very important day—your birthday!

What are the messages in your family about the holidays? Are they positive or negative? Do the holidays make you happy? Sad? Lonely? Miserable? Uptight? Anxious? It is often said that the holidays are the loneliest time of the year for thousands and thousands of people.

Whatever memories or feelings you come up with, you can make a change, starting now, about how you will experience all future holidays and birthdays. Let yourself feel *everything* that comes up for you concerning holidays, and feel free to write and talk about it. You may think that looking at your feelings about holidays may be trite or unimportant, but I see many people every year who are deeply affected by the holidays. So don't feel you have to be victimized by the holidays! You can get free from all the old garbage.

JOURNAL WORK

Exercise 1
Areas of Stress

Divide a page in your journal into two columns of approximately equal sizes. Label the left column "My Stresses," the right one "Where I Hold The Stress."

Think about areas of your life where you are feeling particularly stressed: money, other people, job, school, children, parents, brothers or sisters, illness, weather, car trouble, commute problems, etc. Write down everything that causes you to feel stressed. As you are writing, notice how your body is feeling. Are any aches and pains rearing their little heads? Are you becoming aware of a pain that has been there for quite a while? Would you write down whatever awareness you are having about your body?

Exercise 2
Evaluate Your Depression Level

If you feel you may be suffering from depression, or have occasionally gone through bouts of depression in the past, use the Beck Depression Inventory to evaluate yourself. If you find that you score between 10 and 23, repeat the inventory in two weeks. If your score is still within that range or is even higher, consult with a physician, preferably a psychiatrist who is skilled in the treatment of depression. Remember, depression is one of the most common illnesses seen by doctors, and there are effective treatment programs that make it completely unnecessary for you to suffer any longer.

Exercise 3

Holiday Word Association

Read over the following list very slowly. When you come across a word that brings up strong feelings of any kind, record in your journal what that word is and what you are feeling. Here is the list:

Thanksgiving	Christmas
Hanukkah	Shopping
Presents	Cookies/candy/holiday treats
Santa Claus	Snow
Money	Parties
Children	Mom/Dad
Christmas Tree	Family gatherings
Hanukkah bush	Traveling
Friends	Sending cards
Receiving cards	Department stores
Traffic/parking	Expectations you have of others
Recent painful holidays	

Exercise 4

The Way I'd Like It to Be

Ask yourself how you would like holidays and birthdays to be. What changes would you like to make for future holidays or birthdays?

CHAPTER 18

What You Deserve

Help me take the blinders off my eyes and see myself clearly.

—JOHN

Let's look at the word "deserve." I have seen this little seven-letter word mess up more people! I would love to see it taken out of our vocabulary. Webster defines it as "to be worthy of. . . ." It gives one a feeling of someone always lurking around us, watching our every move, and then, based on our actions and thoughts, *giving us what we deserve.*

If you're good, you *deserve* something good. If you're bad, you *deserve* something bad. It's that simple . . . and that abusive. "To be worthy of." It seems as if it is always hanging over our heads.

Do I deserve happiness?

Have I been good enough to deserve that?

Hey, I don't deserve that!

We deserve to be punished. We're sinners.

Oh, he deserved everything he got.

Be glad that you never got what you deserved.

Are you physically ill right now? Is there a small voice inside that says, "You deserve this illness"? Do you find yourself thinking, "I must have done something wrong to deserve this illness?" Try to answer this question for yourself: Who in your life decides what you deserve or don't deserve? Family members? Friends? Co-workers? Your boss? A religious leader? Your significant other? God? Or you?

Whenever we are judging whether or not we deserve something, we are usually judging ourselves by someone else's standards. My mother might say that I deserve a new coat, while my father might think that I didn't work hard enough to deserve it. This word is about rewards and punishments, guilt and shame. It is about conditional love, which really isn't love at all.

If we have an illness and we believe that we did something to deserve this "punishment," what can we do to get healed? First of all, who decided that we deserved the illness? God? Well, if that's the case, how can you argue with God? If God did decide you deserved to be sick, how could you possibly heal? It's kind of strange if you think about it. If you believe that God gave you the illness for one reason or another, how good can you be feeling about the chances of your recovery? Why would God be inclined to heal you if He had given you this illness as a form of punishment? Can you see what an impediment the concept of being deserving can be to the healing process? In the next few days, pay attention to how many times you think or say the word deserve. Pay attention to how many times others use the word, either about themselves or other people.

No one deserves to be raped. No one deserves to be sick. No one deserves to be poor, or to lose their job. No one deserves loneliness or cruelty or pain!

Don't underestimate the effect of this word in your life. It is important to recognize how you feel about this word and the beliefs you have formed in your mind around it. I can't tell you how many people believe they are sick because they deserve it. I see them every day in my work as a healer.

Before we can get rid of these beliefs and feelings around the word deserve, we need to look at the possible pay-offs we may be getting by holding onto them. By pay-off, I mean a benefit, what psychologists call a "secondary gain." Here are some examples:

BELIEF: I don't deserve to have a loving relationship because I cheated on my spouse.

PAY-OFF: I'll never have to commit to a relationship again—which is something I would like to avoid anyway.

BELIEF: I don't deserve to have nice things in my life because I never take care of them.

PAY-OFF: As long as I hold onto this belief I will never have to work hard enough to get nice things.

BELIEF: I always cheat on my diet, so I don't deserve to be thin.

PAY-OFF: Knowing I'm going to do it anyway, I won't bother to try to change things. Besides, that way I won't ever have to look at why I feel a need to be overweight.

BELIEF: Because I am a sinner, I don't deserve happiness.

PAY-OFF: As long as I hold onto this belief, I will never really have to open up to life and take risks.

How do we start living our lives free of the concept of being deserving? Here's what you can do. First, ask your Higher Power to help you become willing to give up the pay-offs. You need to become willing to get unstuck. When you feel an inner willingness to move forward, which may or may not happen right away, then ask your Higher Power to heal those negative beliefs. That's right. Simply ask that they be healed, which also means that they will be removed. Sound too easy? Do you have a difficult time believing that you deserve it to be that simple? Give that up, too! Be willing to move forward *now*.

JOURNAL WORK

Exercise 1

What Role Does "Deserve" Play in Your Life?

What happened to you that made the whole concept of being deserving seem so real in your life? Is this word a bogeyman to you? Focus your attention on this word over the next few days and ask yourself what you think and feel about it. Does it affect the way you feel about your life? How? Do you hold old beliefs such as, "You deserve disaster, heartache, punishment of one sort or another?" Listen to this voice's responses when you simply think about the word deserve. If you are sick right now and you believe that God gave you this illness because of something you did, how does that affect your relationship with God?

After a few days of simply thinking about these things and observing your reactions to the concept of being deserving, write down your observations in your journal.

Exercise 2

Your Inner Child's Report

Ask your inner child what she/he feels it deserves. What associations does it have with this word? Ask it to record its responses in your journal, using your nondominant hand.

Exercise 3

Your Critical Parent's Comments

Write down in your journal any comments that surfaced from your critical parent while your inner child was writing down what she/he felt about this concept of being deserving.

SECTION II

The Solutions

SECTION II

Contents

SECTION II

Solutions

The wisdom of nature can give us all the answers to our day-to-day problems and show us the way to heal ourselves.

—GERALD G. JAMPOLSKY, M.D. AND DIANE CIRINCIONE

If you are anything like me, you are anxious to discover the quickest solutions for any problem or question. But the first thing I have to tell you is not to be in too much of a hurry. At the same time, don't lose your passion to get better. You are already on your way. You've realized that something isn't right inside, and you are reading books about healing.

Your mind and body are in the process of shifting from the old way of thinking, feeling, and being into a new way—and the key word here is "process." I've always hated that word. It means there are going to be different stages, and that relief from the pain is going to take time. This is simply a fact of life that we must accept on the healing journey.

Asking God, the Universe, or the Higher Power of one's choice for help is very important. Simply ask each day that you continue to have the strength, courage, and desire to grow out of the old pain and into freedom. Many of us get stuck because we lack courage. We fear change and the unknown. Who will we be, once we get rid of the old stories, the old way of thinking and reacting?

We worry that people won't like us anymore if we turn in our victim roles to find freedom for ourselves. You may have already encountered people who will do everything they can to keep you the way you are even though you want to change. Your getting well may very well threaten those closest to you. But you don't need to get caught in this trap.

Make a big sign and keep it close by you. Have it say something like:

This is my journey, my turn for freedom. My time for healing.

It is time to focus on your freedom, peace of mind, and health.

The only way you can really heal is to focus on yourself. Healing your emotions will have a tremendous effect on your body, your mind, your soul, your relationships, your work, your spirituality, your life!

If You're Sick Now

If you have just found out that you are seriously ill, you will want to know what to do. First things first; you scream, yell, and cry until you feel calmer. It may only take five minutes, but you need to express those panicky feelings somehow, or they will affect all of the decisions that you are going to be making about your recovery. You need to be able to express those initial feelings like: "Why me?" "I'm sacred." "I'm mad." "I've been ripped off." "I don't deserve this!" "Why are you doing this to me, God?"

Then you might want to consider the following suggestions:

1. Get a second opinion from a specialist on what your options are.
2. If you have cancer, get the book *Getting Well Again* by O. Carl Simonton, Stephanie Mathes Simonton, and James L. Creighton. Also, call the Simonton Cancer Center in Pacific Palisades, California, or the Cancer Counseling and Research Center in Dallas, Texas. Ask them to send you information about their programs. I have never met the Simontons, but anything that I have ever read by Dr. Simonton feels very right inside.
3. Call Dr. C. Norman Shealy, of the Pain and Health Rehabilitation Center, in LaCrosse, Wisconsin. Again, I have never met Dr. Shealy, but I have heard him lecture. What he says also feels very right. Tell the clinic what you have and ask what they can do for you.
4. Call the Association for Research and Enlightenment (A.R.E.) Clinic in Phoenix, Arizona. Tell them what you are suffering from. Ask them about their program and what they can do for you.
5. If you are interested in alternative treatment programs in Mexico, most of which use a nutritional approach, there is an organization called the Cancer Control Society (CCS) which runs regularly scheduled tours of many Tijuana clinics. This is a private organization that promotes alternative therapies. The current information number for them is: (213) 663-7801. They can also provide

you with a list of people who have gone through these treatment programs with whom you can discuss their experiences.

There are hundreds of noteworthy places to go for excellent treatment. In addition, there are several wellness centers throughout the world. You simply need to ask the Universe to guide you to the right place, and it shall be done!

6. Call one of the *Lifeworks Clinics* (discussed later in this chapter) nearest you to find out when their next clinic is and what you need to do to be enrolled. This four-and-a-half day intensive workshop is designed to look at the underlying emotional issues that are probably the roots of your illness/disease. Chances are that you have been sick for some time, so putting off surgery or whatever physical treatment you need for one more week won't hurt unless your intuition is telling you to have surgery or treatment *now*. In that case, listen to your intuition, go ahead with the prescribed treatment and then do something to address the emotional issues. Just going in and having the problem cut out does not eliminate the emotional roots. If there are emotional issues causing the physical problem, they will manifest themselves somewhere else in the body.

7. Pray for clarification. Ask God, or the Universe, to make your direction as clear as possible. One of the biggest problems I have seen when someone finds out that they're sick is that every friend and relative will have an opinion regarding what that person should do. Or they will have some kind of horror story about what happened to them or an acquaintance of theirs when they came down with the illness you have.

   It's really important to ask your friends and loved ones for lots of love, nurturing, and support, but tell them to keep their stories positive until you have recovered. You don't need to hear their negative stories.

8. Ask God, or the Universe, to put a shield of protection around you so that you are protected from being bombarded with people's fear energy. What that means is that when people find out we are sick, they are afraid. Afraid of how our illness will affect us and our relationship to them. They fear that they will lose us. They worry about all that we will go through. They don't consciously send

those fear thoughts to us, but they often do put them out, and as soon as they are out there we can easily pick them up. We usually have enough fear of our own, so ask for that shield of protection.

9. Go see a competent chiropractor/kinesiologist for his or her opinion on what you should do.
10. Don't abuse your body for letting you down. If your body ever needed your love, it's now. Listen to it. Get a massage. Don't worry about how your body looks. Most massage therapists are concerned about your bones and muscles and aren't concerned with what one's body looks like. Your body is in a crisis! It needs nurturing and understanding.

In spite of my belief that most illnesses have an emotional root, I do not believe that every ache and pain works that way. Sometimes your body is getting rid of toxins, during which you will have flu-like symptoms. You may have an allergy to something, which can account for cold-like symptoms. If the symptoms do not last as long as a cold or the flu, you are probably detoxifying something or you are allergic to something in your system.

If you are sick right now and are searching for some answers, one suggestion I want to convey to you from John is to "surrender to the lessons of the illness." At night, before going to sleep, ask God, the Universe, or your Higher Power to help you surrender to the lessons of the illness. Surrender your fear. Surrender your will. Each morning before getting out of bed, ask God, Universe, or Higher Power to guide you wisely in each decision you make throughout the day concerning your health and well-being.

Personal Therapy

Okay, so what do you do to get on with this healing process, now that you have looked at and written down all of your feelings, beliefs, memories, and pain? First, you ask around to find a competent therapist or clergy-person. If money is a concern, there are still places that will help you. You might have to look a little harder, but they're there. Many therapists have a sliding fee scale, which means that they charge according to your income. Many government offices provide free counseling. Don't sabotage your healing process because of money issues! Ask for help.

Ask friends to recommend someone who is not judgmental or shaming. You need a competent therapist, one who is loving and has been trained to help you unravel all that you have written about yourself in your journal. You need someone who believes that your health problems are connected to emotional issues. You need someone who believes your past does affect your future and who will encourage you to go back and get it all out.

Find a therapist who is relatively busy, who will not hang onto you simply because they need the business. You need someone who will help you as competently and as quickly as possible. A suggestion that always helps me is to ask God or the Universe to direct me to just the right person. You also need to do your part in looking. But you will be amazed at how easily you will be led to the right person if you ask.

Above all, don't let money or pride keep you stuck. Your body's health and healing process should be at the top of your list of priorities! Don't get stuck in what the insurance will or won't pay for. Don't leave your health up to the insurance company. I hear people say all the time, "Well, I'll see if my insurance company will pay. If they don't I just can't afford it." Unfortunately, nearly everyone in the country feels this way, but this is just one more way to be a victim. Please don't let this way of thinking keep you stuck. It isn't as if you can turn this body in and get another one. Get what your body needs in the way of help and slowly chip away at that bill. Bills are a fact of life. They motivate us to go to work, so don't let bills be your excuse for not getting well. This is your healing process.

Once you find a competent, loving therapist, take all that you have written from the exercises and share it with him or her. Sort through it all, feel it, talk it out, and, hopefully, leave all of your pain there. That's the therapist's job. They are like the emotional sanitation department. Dump it all at the emotional garbage station!

When I left my therapist's office each week, I would ask her for an assignment, something that I could work on in between visits. Some of her suggestions I didn't want to do, but I did them anyway. For example, her suggestion that I share one of my feelings each day with at least one person was always a difficult task for me. When I would go into a manic-depressive state, she would ask me to call at least one person each day to help me feel more connected to people and life, rather than continue to feel as disconnected as I had. As I said, I didn't want to do this but I did—and it helped.

Ask your therapist for suggestions for things you can do in between visits, so that you feel your healing process is progressing in the interim. Make a series of appointments, so you can stay in the flow of your healing process.

Good Medical Help

The next part of this process, if you are in physical pain, is to find a good doctor. Do you have one who listens to you and who will spend quality time with you? One who returns your calls? One who treats you with respect? If you don't have a wonderful doctor, it is time to shop around. Don't get caught up in false loyalty. You don't have to go to a doctor just because your parents did or because he or she is your neighbor, etc. Remember, this is your body. It runs like a magnificent machine when all systems are go. When all systems aren't go, you need help! Take your body to someone you really trust. You need someone who will listen to what you have to say.

I wish that the whole world could go to my gynecologist! He's loving. He cares. He's sincere. He's never shamed me for being sick or made me feel that he's too busy for me. Being sick is hard enough without an insensitive doctor telling you that your symptoms are in your head. Please don't think you need to put up with a doctor who makes you feel bad about yourself. There are many qualified physicians out there who went into medicine because they want to help people. Remember, if your body hurts, something is wrong! Don't just wait for days or weeks for the pain to go away. If it persists, your body is talking to you. It wants your attention.

Here are some suggestions concerning doctors and your health. You must fight for yourself! If you are in physical pain, call your doctor or go in to see him or her. If your doctor doesn't return your call, call back. Don't let a nurse put you off. When you do get in to see your doctor, tell him or her all the symptoms that you are having. He or she is not going to know what you "kind of" mean. Your doctor needs to hear the whole story. All of your symptoms. Your doctor's job is to help you fix your body, so you've got to describe what's going on.

Try not to treat the doctor as if he or she is God. Doctors are not God, and giving them that kind of power is just going to get in the way of you getting the help you need. If you happen to find a doctor who wants to be treated like God, go find another one. You're not there to boost his or her ego. You're there for your body's sake. I have heard so many clients say that they don't want to bother their doctor with the pains that they're having or the fears they're experiencing. If the heat went out in your house, would you hesitate to call your local gas company because you don't want to hassle them? If your doctor has a busy schedule, that is not your responsibility. If he is hassled, it's not your fault. Don't get into the "I don't want to be a burden to him or her" kind of thinking. If he is hassled, it is up to him and his office staff to make some changes. It's not up to you. It is their professional responsibility to provide you with the service you require; if they're not doing that it is time for you to find someone who earns their pay.

This is your body. It's your health and your healing process. As I said earlier, you have got to fight for yourself. No one else knows what is going on in your body other than you and your doctor, so keep that line of communication open and take care of whatever it is that you need.

Personally, I would love to see everyone in the world go to a competent chiropractor/kinesiologist at least once a week in the beginning of their healing process. Then start seeing them once or twice a month to maintain good health. Yes, it's true that many insurance companies are not covering chiropractic care, but hopefully the day will come when they will realize its value in preventive health care.

Kinesiology

What is applied kinesiology? It is not a very easy thing to explain. Kinesiologists treat the body as a computer. They believe that the body will tell them accurately, through muscle testing, what is wrong and what is needed. By testing your muscles, they can evaluate your various bodily functions and tell you how the glands, organs, lymphatic system, nervous system, circulation, muscle, and bone structures are working.

I first got involved in kinesiology about seven years ago after quite a bit of resistance. I was afraid that I would have to give up coffee, cigarettes, all of the foods that I loved and would have to live on oats and grains for the rest of my life! I really didn't know a thing about it, except that it was holistic. That made me nervous! They say that everything happens in divine timing, so I guess that I got there when I was supposed to. After seeing how much I have benefitted from it, I wish that I had started it ten years ago.

As you know from reading this book, I have had many physical problems on and off during my life. These have included colon problems, stomach problems, headaches, leg aches, sore back, weak arms from a car accident, poor digestion, allergies, throat problems, and female problems. The list seems endless! It seemed that I was always complaining to someone about not feeling well. I had such a fear that it was all in my head. Severe right-side headaches that persisted for a year finally got me to the kinesiologist's office. My internist had given me pain medication. A neurologist suggested cutting off a cyst that I have on my skull from a car accident. After several tests proved inconclusive, he wasn't sure what else could be causing the problem. I decided to give kinesiology a try. I told myself that I didn't have to go back if it seemed too weird or restricting. It turned out to be quite the opposite!

The chiropractor/kinesiologist spent almost an hour with me in our first session. She didn't tell me to give up all of the foods that I love to eat, nor did she put me on an oat bran diet. She found a weakness in my liver due to toxins in my system. She gave me apple pectin tablets to take for two weeks. The next day, for the first time in a year, I did not have a headache all day! I was impressed.

I started going every other week, because I wanted to feel better. I didn't get any lectures about the evils of coffee or smoking! She told me that as my body continued to get healthy it would just automatically want to give up whatever was causing the problems. That's exactly what happened. When my body was ready to dump the nicotine and caffeine, it slowly and noticeably began losing the desire for both, one at a time. Because I was getting healthier, I believe the process of withdrawal was made a little easier.

After about two years, I felt led to another kinesiologist in Minnesota, whom I have seen ever since. Kinesiology is where I have learned much about the body. It's wonderful! Your body does not lie. It will tell you, through muscle testing, exactly what it needs. If any of the organs are stressed, the muscle testing will tell you what is needed. It also tells you what's going on with your emotions and what needs to be worked on. This is how I discovered the negative effect that feelings and beliefs can have on our bodies.

My body is an open book when I'm with the kinesiologist. He can tell when I've been eating too much of a certain food, or when my body is sloughing off toxins, and what it chemically needs in order to detoxify. When I say chemically, I'm speaking of the natural supplements that help the body through whatever process it is in. Most kinesiologists attempt to work with all three areas of health: structure, chemistry (nutrition), and mentality.

If you have physical problems and have been told by the medical profession that nothing is wrong with you or that you are a hypochondriac, go see a kinesiologist! They treat the whole person. They use no drugs, needles, or painful procedures in diagnosing what's wrong. They can determine your body's specific nutritional requirements through muscle testing.

Here's how muscle testing works. You lie down, sit, or stand and put one arm up in the air. They use finger modes and talk to the body using "finger codes," which simply means that they touch the body lightly in specific areas known to be associated with a physiological system.

The kinesiologist then asks questions that have to do with that particular system while gently pulling on your extended arm. If the answer is a yes, your arm will become weak and you won't be able to resist their tugging. That's how it works! Tom and Carole Valentine have written an excellent book called *Applied Kinesiology* which you might want to read if you are interested in pursuing this approach.

Kinesiology is fascinating. Over and over, I've been amazed at how accurate and helpful it has been in my healing process! One thing I have found in trying different doctors, is that not all kinesiologists work the same way. Some are more willing than others to work with you at the deeper levels where emotional pain resides. If you find a competent kinesiologist but it feels as if you could be getting more help, shop around. At first, you won't know for sure what you're shopping for, but if you trust your intuition it will lead you to the right one.

Don't wait until you are in a major health crisis. Find a competent chiropractor/kinesiologist now and get a tune-up. Do what you can to improve the good health that you already have! Not all chiropractors do kinesiology or even believe in it, for that matter. So when you're checking the yellow pages of the phone book for a chiropractor, note whether or not they do applied kinesiology. Or call them and ask directly. You might also ask your friends if they know of a good kinesiologist. It's becoming more and more popular, so hopefully, you won't have difficulty finding a good one.

Twelve-Step Groups

I've talked about the importance of a personal therapist to help you with all of the emotional issues. I've talked at length about finding a competent doctor to help with the physical symptoms. What we need to look at next is the spiritual needs of your body and soul. It's important that you not try to do all of this work by yourself. Consider getting involved in a support group. The twelve-step programs are a great beginning.

What Are the Twelve Steps?

The Twelve Steps of AA are relatively simple, straightforward guidelines that can help us work through almost any kind of habit or behavior that has us stuck:

1. We admitted we were powerless over alcohol—that our lives had become unmanageable.
2. We came to believe that a Power greater than ourselves could restore us to sanity.
3. We made a decision to turn our will and our lives over to the care of God as we understood Him.
4. We made a searching and fearless moral inventory of ourselves.
5. We admitted to God, to ourselves, and to another human being the exact nature of our wrongs.
6. We were entirely ready to have God remove all these defects of character.
7. We humbly asked Him to remove our shortcomings.
8. We made a list of all persons we had harmed, and became willing to make amends to them all.
9. We made direct amends to such people wherever possible, except when to do so would injure them or others.

10. We continued to take personal inventory and when we were wrong promptly admitted it.
11. We sought through prayer and meditation to improve our conscious contact with God as we understood Him, praying only for knowledge of His will for us and the power to carry that out.
12. Having had a spiritual awakening as the result of these Steps, we tried to carry this message to alcoholics, and to practice these principles in all our affairs.

Twelve-step groups, based on these guidelines, are spiritual in nature. You do not need to be alcoholic to live these steps, as they have been adopted by all kinds of groups with different needs. Check your local white pages in your telephone book for the twelve-step group that sounds as if it would fit your needs best. If you can't find anything listed in the white pages, I would suggest you look up the number for your local Alcoholics Anonymous Central Intergroup Office. They usually have the numbers of other twelve-step groups in their area. Here's the latest list:

Alcoholics Anonymous

Al-anon (spouse or loved one of an alcoholic or drug addict)

Cocaine Anonymous

Codependents Anonymous

Co-Survivors of Incest Anonymous

Emotions Anonymous

Families Anonymous

Gamblers Anonymous

Narcotics Anonymous

Overeaters Anonymous

Parents Anonymous

Pill Anonymous

Recovering Couples Anonymous

Sex Addicts Anonymous

Sex and Love Addicts Anonymous

Sex-aholics Anonymous

Co-Sa (a step group for the loved ones of sex addicts)

Shoplifters Anonymous

Smokers Anonymous

Shoppers Anonymous

Spenders Anonymous

Survivors of Incest Anonymous

Twelve Steps for Christian Living

Twelve Steps for Spiritual Growth

Women for Sobriety

You will want to check the groups out first before going in and telling your whole life story. First, get a sense of how the group feels. Ask for literature. Most twelve-step groups run strictly on $1.00 donations from each member weekly. There are no dues or fees. If you can't afford a dollar, no one will hassle you or judge you. It's strictly voluntary. There are no memberships. There is no test to take in order to get in. As a matter of fact, all that you need is a desire to get better.

The reason for the word "anonymous" is that your anonymity is protected. At true twelve-step meetings everything you say stays at the meeting.

Groups set up by gender (only for men or only for women) can also be really helpful, and I highly recommend attending one. It's scary to sit in with a group of strangers and talk about who you are. But, remember, newcomers are strangers for only a short time. You will learn more about yourself by listening to other people of the same gender talk about themselves. It really works!

Lifeworks Clinics

Lifeworks is a program designed to help discover and work through self-defeating patterns of living. It provides help and a safe environment where you can take a good, hard look at your family of origin—your roots. It is especially helpful for those of us who are: (1) struggling with issues of compulsive, addictive, or self-defeating coping patterns; (2) struggling with codependency and related intimacy issues; (3) adult children of alcoholics or from other types of dysfunctional family backgrounds, and (4) survivors of emotional, physical, and sexual abuse or neglect.

My experiences at a Lifeworks clinic not only saved my life, they changed it from the old, destructive patterns to a freedom that I never thought I would find. They create a unique and safe environment to feel your feelings, to let the inner volcanoes explode if they need to, and feel good about it.

I'm not even going to try to explain the wonderful process they take you through. If you are feeling stuck and are tired of it, I strongly suggest that you find out more about Lifeworks or similar programs in your area. The locations throughout the United States are listed here.

Lifeworks Clinic
National Locations/Contact Agencies

St. Paul/Minneapolis, Minnesota
Friel & Counseling Associates
(612) 482-7982 (main number)

Miami, Florida
Family Passages

Sioux City, Iowa
Gordon Center

Orange County, California
Pathways to Discovery

Dayton/Cincinnati, Ohio
New Life Family Workshops

Texas
Family Recovery, Inc.

Oklahoma City, Oklahoma
Associates in Co-Dependency Treatment

When Was the Last Time You Had a Good Cry?

Crying is an important part of anyone's healing process. It's a way that Nature gave us to release our fears, our hurts, our frustrations, and our pain, whether physical or emotional. It's one of the best ways to cleanse ourselves. Yet, so many of us believe that we can't cry, or we won't allow ourselves to cry.

Many people pride themselves on not being able to cry. I have heard clients proudly say, "I can't cry. I haven't cried in years. I don't remember the last time that I cried. You'll never see me cry. I'll never give so and so the satisfaction of seeing me cry. Crying is for babies." And then there are all the old prohibitions against boys and men crying: "Big boys don't cry. Grown men don't cry." Many of us see crying as a sign of weakness. Many of us are embarrassed by our tears. Some use tears as manipulation. Many of us fear losing control or feeling that vulnerable.

Let me pass something on to you that I learned at the Lifeworks clinic about vulnerability. Most people try to stay in control of their emotions, feelings, thoughts, expressions, etc. so they won't be vulnerable. My therapist said that it's just the opposite. When we are flowing with life, being spontaneous, feeling and expressing our feelings and passion about life, we are being vulnerable. This actually puts us in control. She said that the people who are in control in the sense of sitting on their vulnerability are actually out of control.

The scary part is that it means we need to allow ourselves to express our feelings, our needs, our desires, our thoughts. We need to let go and learn to be spontaneous in our everyday lives and that means if we need to cry, we need to cry *now*.

How do you feel about crying? Do you allow yourself to cry when you feel like it? Do you hold back your tears? Are you afraid of your tears? Your sadness? Your hurt feelings? Do you worry about losing control or being too vulnerable?

I used to be afraid of crying. I felt that if I really let the tears out, I would never stop. I worried that I would lose control. When I got into recovery, my sponsor encouraged me to work on crying. At that point in my life, I was so blocked that I actually had to pray and ask my Higher Power to help me release the blocks to crying. I went to sad movies and played sad songs. It really helped me a lot. Once I started crying, it seemed to come quite easily. I think I had held so much inside for so long. It isn't that I had never cried before. I cried a lot, but I would never just let myself cry it all out when I was confronted with something that made me very sad. I would cry and then tell myself that was enough.

If you are one of those people who won't let yourself cry, I want you to ask yourself why. Don't let yourself get by with an "I don't know." Whatever block you've got about crying, you've got to get past it. The block has to be released so you can get on with this important part of your cleansing process.

Most of us get our messages and attitudes about crying from our parents and their parents. If you can't figure out what your blocks to crying are, maybe you should look at how your family members expressed their sadness or hurt. What messages were you given?

Give these questions some thought and write down in your journal what messages you are carrying around about crying. If you are one of those people who can't or won't let yourself cry, this exercise can be particularly important. If you are a person who does allow yourself to cry, you don't have to write anything down.

Crying is an important part of anyone's healing process. I love it when a client cries during a healing session. These people are doing some terrific releasing, and they usually feel so much better than the clients who fight back the tears during their healing.

If you don't cry because of pride, consider giving up that kind of pride! Ask the Universe for help with being able to cry. The answers will come in dreams, or from a friend, an article in the newspaper, something on the TV or radio. The Universe has a million options to show us how to overcome our blocks.

What have you got to lose from crying? Just lots of old, mothballed stuff that's sitting inside of your body! Who needs that? Ask the Universe to help you cry. It can be a wonderful experience.

Inner Child Dolls

Donna Eitel, who lives in Minneapolis, used to make inner child dolls. She'd have you supply her with a picture of yourself as a child and tell her about yourself at that age. Then she'd create a doll that looked similar to what you looked like in the picture. While creating your doll, she would focus on your character, your personality, your essence. While Donna no longer does this, the idea is a good one and continues to be carried out by individuals around the country.

Having an inner child doll that reminds you of yourself in a certain period of your life can be invaluable with any inner child work you might want to do. Establishing a relationship with your doll, the way you perhaps did with a doll or a pet when you were a child, can help in many ways. You can talk to your inner child (the doll) the way you wished people would have talked to you when you were that age. You can treat the inner child the way you wanted to be treated as a child. Does it sound too silly or simply not possible?

Just before Donna stopped making her dolls, my sister purchased me one to celebrate my birthday. I had wanted one for years, but I always told myself that it was too much of an extravagance. I was delighted when my sister handed me a gift certificate for a "Donna Doll." I met with Donna and brought her a picture of myself when I was three years old. We talked about what I was like as a child—with blonde hair and big brown eyes, kind of shy, smiled a lot, felt afraid a lot, loved my grandfather a lot—like that.

Donna called me a few days later to tell me that my doll was ready. When I got to her house, I looked around her room of dolls to find mine. There on the floor, right in the middle of a bunch of adorable little dolls, was this blonde, brown-eyed doll that I knew, instinctively, was me or should I say, my doll. I felt such a psychic connection to this little doll. I could feel my inner child glowing.

Daily I talk to this very special doll. When I do this, I can feel my inner child responding in a very positive way. At night, I tuck my doll into bed, and it feels as though I'm tucking my inner child into bed. I tell her that she's safe. I tell her that nothing will ever happen to her at night again to cause her to be afraid. I tell her that she's very special, and I can feel my own inner child responding with such joy. I constantly talk to this doll and touch her in a very loving, nurturing way so that my inner child will continually heal. It has become a wonderful part of my healing process.

Both men and women use these dolls. They are for anyone interested in healing their inner child. The little boy dolls are just as wonderful and alive as the little girl dolls. It's very healing to talk to, love, and nurture your inner child in this way. Healing the inner child is a vital part of the healing process.

My doll doesn't look exactly as I did when I was a child, but she does have my essence. If there is someone in your community who is gifted like Donna and makes inner child dolls, I highly recommend that you get one made for yourself as a part of your healing process. If you cannot find anyone doing this in your area, you may wish to buy a doll that appeals to you in the same way, a doll that will represent your inner child.

Laying-On-Hands Healing

Healings such as the kind I do also helps people in their healing process. Laying-on-hands healing is very straightforward. I've been doing it for twenty-five years, and it's so simple, in fact, that most people have difficulty with it for that reason! They try to complicate it with rituals, sounds, methods, step-by-step instructions, etc.—as if God isn't enough!

If you do not know a reputable healer to go to or if there isn't one in your local area, there are three ways that you can receive a healing. For each of the three ways to receive healings, be sure that you first do the following:

1. Sit or lie down in a comfortable position, uncrossing your arms and legs.
2. Ask God or the Universe to clear the area around you of other people's energy, such as worries, fears, negative thoughts, or illness.
3. You may want to play very relaxing music to help your mind switch gears from the fast pace of the day into a relaxed state.

Suggestion No. 1

The first suggestion for receiving a healing is to lay your hands on your body. Anywhere will be fine. Ask God, or the Universe, or your understanding of a Higher Power to send healing energy through your hands to heal your body.

Suggestion No. 2

The second way to receive a healing is to keep your hands to your side and ask God, the Universe, or your Higher Power to channel a healing to you. You may feel a hand pressing on you, or you may not.

Suggestion No. 3

Third, ask someone close to you to lay their hands on you (in a nonsexual way). Then have them ask God, the Universe, or their Higher Power to channel the healing energy through their hands.

In all three situations you may feel heat, a tingling sensation, or a sensation like mentholatum or other aromatic salve flowing through your body. This is the healing energy. Everyone is capable of channeling healing energy.

My first book, *Hands That Heal*, gives complete instructions for channeling healing energy. You may want to purchase a copy to read more about this subject, but for now my suggestion is to keep it simple. Remember, you are simply the channel for the healing energy. God is the healer. You need do nothing but provide the vehicle for this to happen. Don't try to intellectualize the process. Let the universal healing energy flow through your hands.

Healings usually require between twenty and forty minutes, depending upon the needs of the body. When you have finished the healing, run your hands in a circular, counter-clockwise motion over the area where your hands were placed. Do this circular motion about ten times. This places a protective shield on the body.

You can receive a healing as often as your body will receive the energy. If you are physically sick, I would recommend once or twice a day. If you are not physically sick but want to maintain good health, a healing once or twice a week is usually a good idea.

t.t.G.

Another solution I especially like is to t.t.G. (talk to God). I don't even want to say the P-word (prayer) because so many people these days get stuck there. They see the word and immediately stiffen up and think of some formalized, ritualistic prayer they learned as a child.

I don't believe God wants to hear some formalized prayer. I believe God wants to hear from you. Your thoughts, feelings, needs, desires, wants, fears, tears, and anxieties. I believe that whatever you have to say, God wants to hear it!

You are not alone on this journey. Hopefully, you've got a good therapist, you're seeking a good chiropractor, or at least you have a good doctor whom you can rely on for physical problems. Possibly you're attending a support group, but there's still more help available to you . . . t.t.G. (talk to God) and l.t.G. (listen to God).

When I first got into recovery, the idea of talking to God was a little scary for me, as it is for a lot of other newcomers to a spiritual way of life. At my church, someone came up with the idea of a God Box. Whenever any of us had a need to talk to God or had a prayer request, we would write it down and put it in the God Box. The youth group at our church has a God Can. I like that idea better than a God Box because it's a reminder that "God can."

Writing letters to God has become a great way for me to share with Him all that goes on with me. It's also a good way to get to know myself. I have saved my letters to God throughout the years, and it's fun to look back at them and see my progress. It's also been a good way to build faith and to see that the prayers do get answered.

Fortunately for me, not all prayers are answered with a yes, including things that I thought I just had to have, such as relationships with men, certain jobs, or places to live. I have learned that what I think I must have is sometimes not that good for me in the long run.

Step eleven of the Twelve-Step Program says: "We sought through prayer and meditation to improve our conscious contact with God as we understand Him, praying only for knowledge of His will for us and the power to carry that out."

I have learned, after some resistance, to pray for knowledge of God's will for me. This has always turned out to be better than my will for myself. Sometimes my issues about unworthiness and undeservingness get in the way. What I want or see for myself often comes up short of God's will for me.

There was a man in my life with whom I really wanted a relationship. I begged and pleaded with God to please let it happen. I was sure that man was all I needed to be happy and feel complete. This went on for two years. We would date, but as soon as we would get close, he'd go away physically and emotionally. I couldn't see how bad he was for me. I look back at all of those old, pleading prayers. Thank God I didn't get what I thought I had to have! God has always had something better in mind, so I have come to a place in my prayers where I ask for God's will to be done. This doesn't mean that I don't ask for my desires, dreams, wants, and needs, but because experience has taught me that God's will is much greater, I always end my requests with, "Thy will be done, not mine." That way, I've said what's on my mind and still sought my highest good!

People often ask me how I pray. Some seem surprised that I talk to God as I would my best friend. I need God to know me. I need to feel that connection to my source. That oneness. All throughout the day, I talk to God about everything: decisions that need to be made, feelings that I have, fears that I bump up against. I ask for guidance all the time. No, I don't get down on my knees. I used to, but I don't think that it matters to God what position I'm in when I'm talking to him. I think that what's most important is the communication. It helps me feel grounded, centered.

I prefer to t.t.G. before I get out of bed in the morning. Sometimes, however, I get going so fast because of an appointment that I don't take the time to check in. About 10:00 in the morning, I start feeling pretty scattered. I'm not clear about my day. When it hits me that I didn't take the time to t.t.G., I go and sit some place by myself, away from people, TV, and radio, and check in. "Good Morning. What do I need to do today or know about today? Please help me plan my day so I don't waste time or energy. Please guide me continually." If there is something specific that I need help with, I include that in my conversation with Him. Once I'm done with t.t.G., then I l.t.G., which I'll talk more about next.

I think that it's so important to our daily peace of mind and sense of direction to talk to God. I can't imagine the chaos if I were trying to figure this out all by myself. What about you? How comfortable are you with talking to God? If you haven't talked to God for a long time or if you have never talked to Him, don't let that stop you! God didn't go away. God doesn't hold grudges or keep score. God is there for you to talk to about yourself, your life, your troubles, your dreams. Whatever concerns you, concerns God.

Some of you may only feel comfortable talking to God by starting out with a ritualistic, formalized prayer. That is fine, but please don't stop there! Keep talking about who you are and what you need to talk about. I know that if you haven't done this for a while, it can be scary or feel strange. Just go slowly. Be gentle with yourself. Tell God that you're afraid, nervous. Every day try to make some conversation. After awhile, you will sense the presence of God. The feeling of God. You'll know God's listening. As time passes, you'll talk more and more. Developing this relationship is a process, just like everything else. Just start . . . talking to God . . . and when you're done talking, go on to the next step, l.t.G. Listen to God!

I.t.G.

After you spend time talking to God, you need to give God some time to talk back. Praying is talking to God, or the Universe, and meditating is listening to God or the Universe. Meditation is a means by which our minds and bodies become calm. The purpose is to get your mind off the outer world and focus on your inner world—that inner sanctuary. While it may seem impossible at times to become calm, it really isn't! There are wonderful meditation books on the market, or meditation classes you can attend. Many bookstores also carry cassette tapes that you can listen to that will teach you how to meditate. At first, I would caution you to *keep it simple.*

You need to take yourself away from the "busyness" of the world and become still. Even if it's just for five minutes. Some people have a special place set up in their homes or offices where they meditate. Some need to go to a church or a meditation center. Some like to meditate in a natural setting, such as a garden, a park, the woods or seashore. Remember, whatever works for you is right. Personally, I don't have a specific place set up for meditation. In the mornings, before I climb out of bed, I lie there in that very relaxed state and ask God what I need to know or do for that day. Images come to me. So do feelings. Inspirations, too, of people to call or places to go. Direction. Throughout the day, I keep one ear open to the world and one ear open to God. Someone said in a sermon, "God doesn't shout . . . God speaks softly, so don't expect your guidance to come thundering in from on high. Keep an open ear to God at all times." God speaks to us through our intuition. If we don't pay attention to our intuition, the answers come in other ways, like our thoughts, our friends, family members, and others. You might feel an inner nudge to go to the grocery store, and that's where you will find the answer that you've been looking for. Our answers come in so many ways. God certainly isn't limited in how He can get answers to us. That makes it fun!

It is important to try each day to connect with our source. It helps us feel less crazy and scattered and more centered. The problem with meditation is that people think it has to be more complicated than it is. Simply put, it is taking the time to listen to the Universe, God, our Source, or whatever you want to call it, so that we feel centered and directed. It may be easier in the beginning to focus on something other than yourself, so I suggest getting a tape or meditation book. Listen to the tape or read the book for that day. Focus or meditate on those words during that day. Periodically, throughout the day, think back to the words of your meditation. Become calm again. As I said earlier, throughout the day I check in with my Higher Power for any new direction that I may need to get.

Some people get so intimidated by the word meditation that they never try it. They are afraid they won't do it right. Don't get caught up in that. Just take some time each day to focus on your source—whatever you call your Higher Power. Talk and then sit in the silence and listen. Don't worry if nothing comes; there's always tomorrow!

Affirmations

Affirmations are positive statements that can help to change the way we view ourselves or the world around us. Most people, upon discovering that they are holding onto negative beliefs, try to change these by saying affirmations several times a day. For example:

Negative Belief	*Affirmation*
I am fat.	I am thin.
I don't deserve love.	I deserve love.
I am afraid of snakes.	I like snakes.

Through the use of repetition, affirmations can create a pattern of positive thinking in the mind. My concern with affirmations has to do with something that Reverend Philip Laporte of the Unity Church, Bloomington, Minnesota, said in one of his sermons:

> *"Messages of years past are very important to be aware of. If we are affirming what we want, but we have these messages and beliefs from the past, the results can be very mixed."*

In order to change existing thinking, it's important first to understand what those beliefs really are!

If you are overweight and have a belief that says, "You will always be fat because it is hereditary," all of your affirmations that "I am thin" aren't going to change that belief! The results are going to be mixed. The belief and affirmation will wrestle with each other over which is going to come out on top. So, if we have been saying affirmations but not getting the results we desire, we may have to go deeper in order to uncover beliefs that are getting in the way. Our bodies aren't stupid. They have a wisdom we can't fool with all our affirmations.

Think about it this way: If you feel overweight, but every day you repeat the affirmation "I am thin," your body is just going to feel confused. How can she trust such a statement when she knows it's not true . . . she really isn't thin. Similarly, if we are in financial trouble and are saying affirmations that "I am prosperous," there is going to be a huge credibility gap that your body and mind are going to pick up. The same goes for affirmations like "I am beautiful" or "I am healthy" when they are obviously not true at the present moment.

For affirmations to work well, we have to acknowledge what is true right now and allow that truth to be reflected in the positive statement. Thus, you might also say, "I am now in the process of becoming prosperous," or "I am in the process of feeling and being attractive," or "I am in the process of becoming healthy."

Affirmations are very helpful whenever you are trying to change something in your life. But you need to say your affirmations every day, twenty to thirty times a day. Some people say them in the morning, at noon, and at night before they go to sleep.

Respect your body's intelligence. It knows what's going on. You can't expect change to occur if you just say your affirmations each day but continue to act in the same old way. You've got to implement the necessary changes to bring about those positive changes. Examples of the wrong way to do this would be the person who munches on a Dove Bar while repeating affirmations that she is losing weight, or who purposely puts herself deeper in debt while affirming that she is becoming prosperous.

Along with making positive affirmations, take whatever action you must to bring the new reality into being. If you want to lose weight, eat less. If you want to be more prosperous, look for more money-making opportunities or look for ways of expanding your present business or profession. As your thinking changes, you will find yourself automatically doing more and more to ensure the outcome you desire.

If things don't begin to change after three weeks or so, the chances are that you are holding onto a negative belief that is preventing you from moving forward. For example, you might find that your body doesn't want to be thinner because putting on weight was once its way of protecting itself from physical or sexual abuse. If you are not prospering, you might be holding onto a belief that you shouldn't be wealthy because then you would have to be more responsible for your own life. If you continue to feel unattractive, perhaps it may be because your present way of being allows you to be invisible, providing a sort of camouflage so others won't notice you.

You will find that positive affirmations, joined with actions that support them, become most effective the moment you are able to get your negative belief systems out. The journal work in Section I, particularly Chapter 3: Negative Feelings and Beliefs, is an excellent place to begin.

Choices

Emmanuel says in *Emmanuel's Book II: The Choice of Love*, "The minute you say, there is another way to do this, you have found the other way!" In order for us to see other choices or solutions, we need to be willing to let go of being victims. Thinking like, feeling like, and believing that I am a victim has been one of the most difficult beliefs that I have had to work out. It is so much easier to point the finger at other people in my life and say, "It's your fault that I am the way I am," or "It's your fault I'm having a bad day," or, "If only my spouse would get his act together, then I would be happy."

It's been difficult for me to admit that I play and wear the victim role very easily. It seems so automatic to start blaming as soon as something goes wrong. Why is it so much easier to point a finger of blame than to take responsibility for what happens in our lives? I think that a big part of it comes from so many of us being afraid of making mistakes. To have to admit that we made a mistake can sometimes be more than we feel we can do.

I have a friend who chooses to believe the negative side of everything. He says that then he won't be discouraged when life lets him down. I know there are plenty of people who live by that same philosophy. Unfortunately, when life is good to them, they seem disappointed too. That's how it is with my friend. Whenever something wonderful happens in his life, he can barely talk about it. When he finally does share the good news, he ends the story with, "We'll see." This usually means, "We'll see if it is really going to be good. We'll see if this really isn't just a hassle wrapped in a pretty package. We'll see if life isn't just messing with me."

A few years ago, my best friend died from lung cancer. Whenever anything positive happened in her life, she would always give me this certain look and say, "We'll see." She would never just let herself bask in the positive experience. She was always afraid of being let down.

One thing that I have learned about life is that it invariably gives me what I'm expecting. It's true. I may be praying for a new car but if I am expecting to get a used car with lots of mileage, that's what the Universe will deliver. It seems to go back to those beliefs again! What we believe to be true is how it's going to happen.

A Slip of the Tongue Leads to New Understanding

Most of us have heard the saying, "I'll believe it when I see it." But a few years ago, while talking to my minister, I made a slip of the tongue and said, "I'll see it when I believe it." We both had a good laugh with that one! But there was also an important truth expressed in my mistake. Our beliefs really do tend to determine what we see! If I believe that work is going to be crummy, it will be crummy. If I believe I'm going to gain weight, I will. If I believe I'm never going to get a vacation, I won't. Have you noticed how the power of belief works in your life?

The good news is that once I changed my belief that I had to be a victim, life itself changed. And as life changed, it went right around in a circle and supported my new beliefs. Honest! All you need is a willingness to turn in your victim's role and start to look for choices. Yes, choices! Every situation in life has at least two choices. Some have more.

Sometimes it's difficult to see the choices in a situation, particularly if it's painful. I want to pass on to you something that a close friend, Virginia Miller, told me. She said that whenever you are in a situation that you don't like or don't want to be in, *thank it*! Thank the experience!

Sounds a little bizarre, doesn't it? But here's an example of what I mean. I was in a relationship with an alcoholic. It was very painful. This man was determined not to quit drinking. I was in the beginning stages of recovery from drinking and was a little shaky myself. Ginny said to me, "Echo, you've got to thank God for this experience." She said to thank the experience a hundred times a day, if that's what it would take for my pain to begin to ease. She said that even if my heart wasn't in it, I should thank God, thank the experience.

After a few days of half-heartedly doing this, my attitude started to change. I was seeing the experience in a different way. For instance, I started to see clearly how I had become lost in this man's alcoholism. I had lost myself because I totally focused on him. I realized I had to get back to myself and work on my own twelve-step program. I wanted to live differently. I slowly began to see how destructive the relationship was and to let him go. This was something that I had tried to do previously, but without success. Changing my attitude about that experience, the pain, the frustration, the powerlessness, giving thanks for the knowledge that I was learning—all these together helped me to heal that period of my life.

Many, many times over the years, when I have been in emotional pain, Ginny has lovingly reminded me to thank the experience until I feel peace inside. Can you see how doing this gets you to focus on the positive side of any situation? Simply give it a try and let yourself experience how it works.

When I was younger, my mom taught me to always look for the good in every situation. There have been many times when that's been pretty tough, but it sure is a blessing when you can do it! If we are in prison—whether literally or at our jobs, in our relationships, with our health, or with our addictions—we can set ourselves free every day with our own attitudes. We just need to be willing to see things differently.

The attitude we bring to the world each day is a twenty-four-hour choice. We can choose to be snarling, crabby, hateful, spiteful, downright nasty, or we can try to look at the whole situation in a different light. If you have the attitude that you choose your experiences in order to learn and grow, things will not be so glum. You will be excited about all of the possibilities for growth and learning. And you'll stop seeing them as static events that will never change, seeing them instead as opportunities that can reveal a new direction.

Unfortunately, most of us can't see the choices that are in each situation. For example, let's look at a work situation, where the boss or fellow employee drives you crazy. The two of you may get into power struggles every day—a "who's right, who's wrong" sort of thing. Did it ever occur to you not to get into it in the first place? You don't have to fix blame one way or the other. You can walk away and bless the person or situation. I know that this may be the last thing you want to do, but try it anyway. When confronted with such lessons, just ask yourself this single question, "Would I rather be right or be at peace?" The results can be amazing!

If changing your attitude and blessing the situation doesn't help, then it is time to come up with another choice. Don't tell me that you have no choice. Life never gives us only one choice. I know there are some situations that seem incredibly bleak, as if there is no other choice, but life is too creative only to offer us one choice! And if life doesn't appear to offer a choice, create one for yourself. This goes back to being willing to let go of being a victim. Yes, as helpless children we are thrown into many situations in which we have no choices. We are at the mercy of others. As adults, we can use our creative energy to come up with choices and solutions which as children we simply couldn't even imagine.

If you have something going on in your life and can't find a different solution or choice, let me give you a couple of suggestions: (1) Write down the dilemma and look at it as objectively as possible. Think of it as your best friend's problem, not yours. See what choices you could come up with then. (2) Write down your problem. Hand it to your best friend. Ask what choices he or she sees as solutions.

Being a victim or feeling like one, is like going through life in a straitjacket. Your arms are tied, so you have no way of protecting yourself. You're dependent on other people to bail you out when you get into trouble. It's a terrible way to live! This is your life and you have every right to experience all of the goodness that life has to offer! You are the only one who can prevent this with your attitudes, beliefs, limitations, fears, self-doubt, anger, hatred, etc. You can stay stuck forever, or you can start asking, "Is there another way to do this . . . ?" That's when the journey really begins!

New Age Movement

For some of you, this book may be your first introduction to the New Age movement. If so, you may be wondering exactly what the term "New Age" means. I would imagine that if you asked ten different New Age practitioners what they thought the movement was, you would get ten different opinions. Despite this, we would all be saying basically the same thing. Some describe New Age as new thought, but in reality it often has to do with very ancient thought.

Back in the 1960s, the Beatles brought to the attention of the modern world many ancient teachings from the East. That was when many of us first heard about meditation. Unfortunately, many people associate gurus, meditation, going within, looking for oneself, and seeking the "truth" with pot smoking and flower children. This is unfortunate, since it has left many people fearful of the New Age.

To me, New Age is about spirituality, developing a close personal relationship with a Higher Power of our choosing—not blindly accepting the relationship with God that organized religion taught us as children. So many people today are searching inside for that Higher Power, rather than accepting the old ideas of an unreachable God who sits on a throne up in Heaven. Jesus spent his adult life giving us the tools that we require to live a spiritual, loving, and abundant life. Today many people are feeling an emptiness inside that they are trying to fill with every conceivable material thing that they can get their hands on. To me, that search for an "inner knowing," to know ourselves and our Higher Power, is what the New Age is all about. It's getting away from looking at life only through the intellect; it's connecting with and trusting our intuition, our inner knowingness.

Another word that comes to mind to describe the New Age is "alternatives." There are many health care alternatives that are discussed in Appendix A. These alternatives are choices that we can make outside the medical profession, which typically treats only symptoms. Health problems are treated in a more holistic way by professionals within the New Age movement. For example when a body is physically sick, a health care practitioner looks at the whole person to sum up what could be causing the problem. In addition to examining the physical problems, an alternative health care professional also looks at what's going on emotionally, mentally, and spiritually. When I refer my clients to a New Age doctor, I am referring them to a doctor who will address all of these areas, not just from the point of view of mainstream medicine.

I would describe the New Age as a movement of personal empowerment with a global viewpoint. New Age doctors treat the whole person, building on strengths rather than focusing on weaknesses. New Age churches teach us about our own divinity while teaching us how to relate to a Higher Power. New Age teachers teach us how to go within ourselves to find the serentity of the Kingdom of Heaven. It's no longer other people telling us to worship them or their version of their God. Rather, these teachers show us how to find our own connections with a Higher Power, to know our minds and our hearts, bodies, and souls. Thus, we are empowered to find the missing pieces, to embrace the child within, and to celebrate our divine stature as children of God.

While I believe that New Age thought is not new, I do believe the movement itself is new—within the last twenty years. Yet, a dear friend claims that the New Age began with the birth of Christ! Today, there are New Age magazines, music, books, talk shows, columns in the newspapers, etc. The movement is growing out of our own deep, inner knowing, which says to each of us that there's more to life, God, and self than we've been led to believe. People involved in the New Age are searching for answers. The good news is that they're finding what they are searching for. This can be a very exciting journey. Clearly, the New Age is not about pot smoking or flower power. It's something that's real and dynamic; missing pieces are being filled in. Being on a spiritual journey isn't always easy. It demands a lot of each person, to clean ourselves out and make us whole. That's what it's all about—going from having holes to being whole.

A Word of Caution

I do need to add a word of caution here about some New Age practitioners. Not everyone that you will meet along the way is on a spiritual path themselves. Yes, there are wolves in sheep's clothing in these professions, as in any other.

Recently, I received a call from a woman who had a psychic reading in Minneapolis. Her psychic went by the title of Reverend. She said that at the end of the reading he hugged her very tightly and began kissing her on the neck. He had mentioned to her during the psychic reading how he psychically worked his way into people's lives, eventually taking them over. This, of course, scared her! In addition, he called her for the next few days, saying that he wanted to see her again. Her statement to me was, "You people are supposed to be on a spiritual path!"

I believe most of the people who are involved in the healing arts in one form or another are on a spiritual path and truly want to be helpful in your healing process. But there are some who are not sincere and have something other than your best interest in mind. Yes, it can be difficult discerning who is on a spiritual path and who isn't, but don't get discouraged.

Here are some suggestions to help you in your search for the help that's right for you. First of all, your intuition will help you. Ask your inner voice if "so and so" feels right. If you are not at the stage where you feel confident in knowing what your intuition is saying, here are some other suggestions:

Suggestion No. 1

When looking for services from any health care practitioner, New Age or not, ask your friends if they know anyone that they would recommend. This goes for psychics (tarot card readers, palmists, channelers, mediums), astrologers, healers, massueses, chiropractors, osteopaths, numerologists, herbalists, acupuncturists, Rolfers, shamans, or handwriting analysts, as well as medical doctors and psychotherapists. You may think people would be shocked to find out you are looking, but chances are that some of the people in your life believe in health care alternatives. It's best to go to someone you are referred to, rather than to someone you find in a newspaper.

When I first began my healing and psychic practice full-time in 1978, my intuition told me not to advertise in the newspapers. I couldn't understand why not! How else was I going to get business? It was tough getting started, and my intellect was really pushing me hard to advertise in the papers. My inner voice continued to say no!

One day I asked the Universe to show me clearly what I was to do. The next day I got a letter from a well-respected psychic in our community who said that she had heard through the grapevine that I was now a psychic and a healer. The only advice that she had was not to advertise in the newspapers! She said God would send me clients and if I was sincere in my work my business would naturally grow. I have run my business by her words ever since and have done very well. (Thanks, Mary!) While I'm sure that there are good practitioners out there who advertise, I maintain that if people are good at what they do, they won't have to advertise for a long time. They will naturally attract all of the clients that they need.

If you do see an advertisement in the paper from some practitioner and you don't have any friends who are involved in this community, you can check these people out in a couple of ways: (1) Call your local New Age bookstore and ask if they have ever heard of them; (2) Call a New Age church and ask if they have ever heard of them. You could also look up the Spiritual Frontiers Fellowship or Edgar Cayce's Association for Research and Enlightenment in your area telephone book. I mention these two organizations because they have been around for a long time. Both have chapters throughout the country with good reputations. Also, you could ask them for referrals to wellness practitioners.

Another thing you can do is interview the person over the telephone. Ask questions about what he or she does. How long has he or she been doing it? Listen to the answers with your intuition. Don't assume anything. Take, for example, psychics. Most people assume that we are all the same, that we all work the same and have similar beliefs. Some people still think we dress weirdly and have cats running all over our houses (some do, of course!)

Psychics are each gifted in their own way. Some are clairvoyant, which means the information they get comes in the form of pictures, images, or visions. Others are clairaudient, meaning they "hear" the psychic information they get. Still others are clairsentient, which means that they "sense" the information they receive.

Some psychics read cards, tea leaves, even coffee grounds. Some read past lives, or only see the future and not the past. Others use astrology or numerology to aid them in their work. Some only read palms, eyes, or feet. Spirits can be "channeled" from the other side, which could mean a couple of things: (a) the medium, or channel, goes into a trance and lets an entity or soul of a deceased person enter and use their body to bring messages to others; or (b) the medium or channel opens himself or herself up to an entity or soul of someone on the other side. The entity uses this person's body to channel information, but the medium stays completely conscious of what is happening. This is termed a semi-trance.

I would like to insert a word of caution here. For a while, channeling was definitely the *in* thing for the New Age community. We got some wonderful messages from entities such as Ramtha, Emmanuel, and Lazaris. People were flocking to hear channeled messages sent by spirits from the other side. I mention these three entities because I have learned some wonderful things from all of them and am grateful for their messages. The danger has come from people believing that any spirit from the other side must have all the answers. People then give their power away and live by the words of these entities.

Don't assume that channeled information is always coming from a wise, all-knowing spirit. If you are listening to information channeled from an entity on the other side, listen with your intuition in order to know if it is accurate or not. Sun Bear, a Native American teacher who recently died, used to tell the story about one of the entities from the other side that offered him advice. Every time Sun Bear followed this entity's advice, it would turn out badly. So Sun Bear went to an elder whom he respected and trusted. After hearing the problem, the elder turned to Sun Bear and told him, "Dead don't make you wise."

When I first got into this business of psychic and spiritual enlightenment, I was very naive and gullible. I believed anything that anyone told me, which is why I believe God sent me the teacher that He did. She taught me what was right and good and what wasn't. What you can do is to ask the Universe to direct you toward the right teachers and information. Ask God or the Universe to protect you from the negative craziness that can go on in this community. Ask and it shall be done.

You do not have to be a victim of the so-called New Age practitioners, or any other practitioners, who are not on a good and right path.

Ask around. Check them out intuitively and with your community. Being in your healing process is the most important work you will do in this lifetime. You deserve to have the best help along the way.

Suggestion No. 2

Stay away from anyone who tries to make you feel guilty or shamed.

Suggestion No. 3

Avoid anyone who intuitively feels bad or negative to you, no matter how popular or well-known he or she may be.

Suggestion No. 4

Stay away from anyone who tries to impress you with their own power. No one is more powerful than God. Whenever someone makes you feel anxious, ask God, or the Universe, for protection. See yourself surrounded in a glowing, shimmering white light of protection, knowing that nobody can enter your space unless you allow them to.

Suggestion No. 5

If anyone makes sexual advances, report them to the authorities. Another suggestion is also to report this to your local New Age bookstore and to all of your friends. Don't keep quiet about it! Sexual abuse is known to occur in just about every profession, New Age or mainstream. Knowing that it isn't right and that you have a right to protect yourself from such people should be your first line of defense.

Suggestion No. 6

If anyone says that they cannot help you unless you take off your clothes (except for masseuses or licensed physicians), don't believe them. I have channeled spiritual healing for twenty-five years and have never asked a client to remove clothing. The healing energy works through layers of anything!

Suggestion No. 7

If someone advises you to turn over all of your money or possessions to them, *don't*! Run as fast as you can in the other direction.

Suggestion No. 8

If someone gives you a line about being surrounded by evil spirits and that it would take large sums of money to help or protect you, *don't believe them*! I had a client who had paid a psychic over $5,000 for protection from evil spirits! You don't need to pay anyone hundreds or thousands of dollars for protection.

If you are feeling afraid and want protection, call Silent Unity, a twenty-four hour prayer tower in Lee's Summit, Missouri. They will pray for you every day for thirty days—for free! All you need to do is call [the telephone number is (816) 246-5400] or write them [Silent Unity, Unity Village, Missouri 64065], describing your needs. There are many such prayer services throughout the world. I mention Silent Unity because I have called there many times when I have needed help. It works!

In summary, my suggestion for you when seeking alternatives is to be cautious. Pray for guidance when seeking the help you need. The direction will come; it always does. You do not have to be victimized by anyone. As Kristen Gottschalk Olsen says in her book, *The Encyclopedia of Alternative Health Care:*

> *Information empowers individuals to take more responsibility for their health care. Empowered health care consumers have a sense of themselves and what they want and need. They are open and inquisitive as well as assertive and critical. They demand competence from practitioners who are aware of the effects of any health care session, treatment, or consultation and have a sense of what works or doesn't work for them.*

If you turn to Appendix A on page 229, you'll find brief explanations of the principles behind each of the major types of health care alternatives. For a more thorough explanation of these professions, please consult Olsen's book mentioned above or ask at your local New Age bookstore for other sources of information. Remember, there is no *one* right way to get the healing that you need. Any, or all, of the healing arts could be of use. Just ask your intuition to guide you to the one or several that are right for your needs at this moment.

Intuition

Deep within each one of us is a calming, soft voice that speaks to us throughout the day, giving us accurate advice, direction, and guidance. We aren't meant to guess our way through life. I believe God speaks directly to each one of us through our intuition.

For as long as I can remember, my mother always referred to her intuition as her "intu." She was always saying that her "intu" told her to do this or that. My siblings and I would give her such a bad time about her "intu," but, ironically, it was always accurate. As we grew older, she encouraged each of us to listen to our own intuition. An inner knowingness, she called it.

For me, it took lots of practice to follow my mother's advice. My intellect was always fighting to be in control. I wanted to analyze my inner nudgings. It wasn't until I took a class at Unity Church, in Minneapolis, based on the book *Lessons In Truth* by H. Emilie Cady, that I realized I was doing it all backwards. Dr. Cady says, "Intuition and intellect are meant to travel together, intuition always holding the reins to guide the intellect."

This seemed like an odd idea to me. I hadn't given my intuition that much credit before. When I did listen to it, its guidance was accurate. But I still did not give it much power. When I read in Dr. Cady's book, "Intuition is the open end, within one's own being, of the invisible channel ever connecting each individual with God," I changed my opinion regarding my intuition and inner voice.

That night in class, we had a wonderful discussion about intuition. It was then I realized that intuition is the inner voice of God, always directing us. I began paying much more attention to what I was feeling inside. Shakti Gawain says in her book, *Living In The Light*:

> *It is often hard to distinguish the "voice" of our intuition from the many other voices that speak to us from within: the voice of our conscience, voices of our old programming and beliefs, other people's opinions, fears and doubts, rational head trips, and "good ideas."*

As she suggests, I began "checking in" regularly to hear what my intuition was saying to me. I would ask God a question and then wait for the inner answer. Every time I asked for an answer, something would come, even if the inner voice was telling me to wait, be patient.

I had a hard time giving up the control of my life to this inner voice. My intellect kept thinking it should make all the decisions and come up with the ideas. I went back and forth for years between letting my intellect run the show and letting God, or the Universe, guide me, speaking to me through my intuition. The other difficulty is that most of the world thinks you are crazy if you live by your intuition!

I read Shakti Gawain's *Living In The Light* a year after it was first published. Then for about two weeks, every time I turned around it seemed as if one more person was either telling me about reading the book or about having a feeling that I should read it. The title of the book turned me off. It sounded so New-Age-ish. Little did I know, in my stubbornness, that the book would change my life.

As far as I am concerned, it is the best book written on intuition. If you have not read this book, consider doing so. It will help you connect with your intuition, as well as help in your understanding of your male/female sides, relationships as mirrors, health, money, and the roles that we play. This book has many wonderful things for you to practice in your daily life. It gave me permission to listen to and live by my intuition. Daily now, I ask God for direction or guidance in all matters.

There is a flow that moves through the Universe. It's wonderful to be able to tap into this flow and ride it like a surfer rides a wave. When I do this I feel a sense of oneness with the whole. I check in with my intuition at all times throughout the day. It's an inner feeling of knowingness. Webster defines intuition as "the immediate knowing of something without the conscious use of reasoning."

There have been many, many times my intellect has argued with my intuition. After being very disappointed several times in myself for not trusting that inner voice, I have learned that it is always accurate. Always!

I believe that in order for us to be and stay healthy, we need to trust and follow our intuition. Shakti Gawain writes in *Living In The Light:*

> *If you are willing to allow the Universe to move through you by trusting and following your intuition, you will increase your sense of aliveness and your body will reflect this with increasing health,*

beauty, and vitality. Every time you don't trust yourself and don't follow your inner truth, you decrease your aliveness and your body will reflect this with a loss of vitality, numbness, pain, and eventually physical disease. Disease is a message from our bodies, telling us that somewhere we are not following our true energy or supporting our feelings. The body gives us many such signals, starting with relatively subtle feelings or tiredness and discomfort. If we don't pay attention to these cues and make the appropriate changes our bodies will give us stronger messages including aches, pains, and minor illnesses. If we still don't change, a serious or fatal illness or accident may eventually occur.

When we're not listening to and trusting our intuition it feels like we're trying to swim upstream against the tide. It is an inner feeling of resistance that can be very wearing on our energy. When we are flowing with our inner knowingness, we feel totally alive.

If you are physically sick, you need to quiet yourself and go to that still, small voice within for guidance. You do not need to feel as if you are at the mercy of the health care professionals. Whenever anyone tells you to make a decision about your health care, ask them for all of your choices. Then go off by yourself and ask for guidance. It is difficult to do this when we are faced with a serious health challenge, but the eventual outcome is worth it. This can save you much unnecessary pain and expense. *You will be shown what you need to do.*

Begin *now* to listen to that inner voice. Sometimes it feels like an inner nudging. At first, it is a slight feeling. A soft voice. A gentleness. A "sense" that such-and-such is true. It is your constant source of help.

Begin to do this slowly. Ask for your intuition's help in small decisions, if that makes you feel safer. First, ask your intuition for guidance. When you get a "sense" of the answer, ask your intellect to guide you in implementing that answer. That is how it works! Intuition guiding the intellect!

You need to be patient with this process. Your intellect is likely to say something such as: "Well, we asked for guidance, and nothing came. So let me come up with the answer;" or, "God helps those who help themselves, so we had better do something;" or, "Maybe I should come up with some ideas. We can check them out with the intuition, if you must do it that way."

Your intellect will try its darndest to get back in control! It will constantly remind you that the intuition hasn't given you an answer yet, so maybe just this one time it should come up with the answer. Whenever you need any direction or guidance, ask God or the Universe to help you clearly know what to do—and then be patient. The answer will come.

Forgiveness

"Forgiveness is a process, not an event," according to Terry Kellogg (*The Phoenix,* June 1986). He also says, "As a process, it consists of stages that we move through." I would like to share these stages with you:

Stage 1:

We recognize the wrongs that have been done to us.

Forgetting is not forgiving, and denying the hurt makes it impossible to forgive. This stage is about remembering and then unravelling mysteries around the painful things done to us and the painful experiences we have had.

Stage 2:

We recognize that we have feelings about the wrongs.

Many of us choose to pretend that we don't have feelings about the harm that was done to us. We take the "I don't care" or "I don't feel anything" stance. We try to blot out our feelings with food, drugs, alcohol, shopping, gambling, etc. to distract us from the feelings of hurt, pain, anger, rage, fear, etc. But no matter what we do to blot them out, the fact is that we do have feelings about these hurts and it is necessary to recognize these feelings before we can at last be free of them.

Stage 3:

We embrace the feelings about the wrong.

When I was in the Lifeworks Clinic and first heard Terry say that we had to learn how to embrace our feelings, it scared me. I had spent so much of my life dodging my feelings, and now he was telling me that I had to *embrace* them. He said, "The only path away from our suffering is to embrace the suffering," which originally came from M. Scott Peck's *The Road Less Travelled.* We need to go into the pain. Not just the physical pain, but also the emotional pain!

When I was in the Lifeworks Clinic, my emotional pain was very stuck. I had denied, rationalized, and minimized it for years, so trying to bring it up and feel it was very difficult. We were told that if we were really feeling stuck, to lie down on the floor in a crucifix position, arms and legs spread open, feeling completely vulnerable. They said not to do this alone, so I had two women friends from my group help me in the process. I don't recommend that you do this by yourself, but with a couple of friends that you feel comfortable and safe with, you might give it a try.

Lie on the floor, arms and legs spread out. Ask your body what it is holding in. Images may come; feelings may surface. Whatever comes, *go into it.* Don't resist it. This is how I got the images of all the sexual abuse that I experienced as a child. I cried, yelled, screamed, beat pillows. Whenever I would feel stuck, I'd go back into the crucifix position. My two friends held me when I needed it. They guided me through with questions. They provided a safe environment for me. It was very painful emotionally and perhaps the single most freeing experience in my life. It took less than an hour to release several feelings that I had been storing for years: terror, rage, hate, fear, sadness, emptiness, abandonment, disappointment, loneliness, bitterness, and desperation. I had tried to deny or minimize all of these feelings for years! Why? I was afraid to feel them or to look at them.

Afterwards, I was physically exhausted, but I could feel a sense of newness about my body. My body felt free—literally unstuck. Since that day, I have done more work on embracing the feelings. You can't know what this feels like until you experience the shift in your body's energy once you stop resisting and start embracing the pain. Believe me, it's wonderful!

Stage 4:
We share the feelings with others, sometimes with the wrong-doer him or herself.

Sharing the feelings is sharing the burden. It lessens our feelings of isolation.

Sometimes it helps to share our hurt with the person who hurt us, but you run the risk of being further abused. So this may not be in your best interests. It is certainly not necessary. Most therapists recommend it only when a safe setting can be provided (such as with a therapist) and under only those conditions where the wrong-doer is either in recovery or is willing to work on his or her problems.

Our goal here in this process of forgiveness is to change ourselves, not others. And the change we are seeking is a letting go of the hurt we are holding inside us. The goal of forgiveness is not to let the wrong-doer off the hook or to tell them that what they did is okay. The goal is only to release ourselves from the pain, anger, hurt, and rage which imprisons us.

Stage 5:

We make a decision about what we want to do with our relationship to the wrong-doer.

This usually evolves over time. If the wrong-doer is a family member or friend, we may need to detach from that person for a while. This can mean a period of separation from your own family when the wrong-doer is a parent, grandparent, sibling or other close relative.

This stage may meet with resistance from other family members because it involves a change in how we operate in the system, which will have an impact on the whole family. We often feel guilty for taking care of ourselves rather than everyone else, but just remember, guilt is an integral part of the family dysfunction. It is part of what we wish to heal with forgiveness. A healthy family encourages its members to do what makes them happiest and live where they want to live.

When we allow ourselves to take time away from the wrong-doer for the purpose of healing, we will heal. We will learn healthy boundaries. We will learn what kinds of relationships we want and what we don't want. If and when we come back into the family, it will be under very different circumstances and it will change the whole family dynamic. What usually happens is that you not only change the relationship between yourself and the wrong-doer but you change the relationships of all the family members in some small or large way.

Stage 6:

There will come a sense of serenity and acceptance about the wrong and our relationships with the wrong-doer.

This is the final stage and it does not mean that we no longer have feelings about what happened. There may always be pain or anger at the abuse or neglect. Rather, it means that the feelings we held inside us no longer control us or force us into denial. It means that our relationships no longer suffer from behavior that is inappropriate, defensive, or avoidant.

Sometimes we get stuck at one stage or another and don't complete the process. This lessens the chance for healing the relationship and our lives reflect where we are stuck in our lives.

We also have to be prepared to reenter the forgiveness process as we receive new information or insights into how we've been hurt. Recovery itself is a lifelong process of forgiving ourselves and others. As we do this we become less and less controlled by the past.

The day does come when we have cleaned up all relationships from the past. This includes our relationship with ourselves. Don't stay stuck in blame or hatred. You might as well finish it up this lifetime!

Suicide?

Yes, I'm putting suicide into this chapter, not because I believe it to be a solution, but because some of you may be considering it as a solution! Let me share with you my own experience with this question.

Two weeks before I quit drinking and joined a recovery program, I sat down with a full bottle of Valium and a glass of water. I was tired of the ups and downs, of hopelessness and despair. Alcohol was no longer giving me the lift that I needed. The prescription drugs I was taking seemed to keep me coasting in neutral. But it seemed impossible for me to feel good about life. I just wanted to be free from the pain that I felt.

I sat on my bed, determined to kill myself. As I contemplated doing this, I had a psychic vision of Limbo. I saw many souls there, grieving the loss of their lives, wanting another chance. They were full of despair and hopelessness. A voice told me that this was where I would be going. I was so angry; I didn't want the reality of suicide slapping me in the face like that. I wanted relief, answers, solutions!

I have seen this place called Limbo in many psychic readings when clients ask about a loved one who has committed suicide. Limbo is a place halfway between our earthly plane and Heaven. It's the closest thing I have ever seen, psychically, that resembles what Hell might be like—even though there isn't any fire and brimstone in Limbo. It is full of souls who are stuck in self-pity. This is not a place God condemns us to, should we take our own life. It is our frame of mind that condemns us to Limbo.

One concern that most of my students express when I talk about Limbo is, "Do they have help there?" or, "How come no one is helping them?" They do have help. There are guardian angels to help them out of Limbo and into Heaven, but remember that there was also help for them when they were here on Earth! They chose to ignore this offer of help, and they may choose to continue to refuse it, even in Limbo.

What happens to souls in Limbo? Once they realize their ways were not solutions and they become willing to try something other than their own solutions to their problems, to let go of their strong wills, and to surrender to other solutions besides physical death, they begin to notice there are higher spirits there offering them a way to the white light of heaven. They become willing to reach out, and in doing so, help is on the way. It's about surrendering our strong will.

Once we accept that suicide can't relieve our inner pain, we become open to seeing other solutions to the pain in our present life. That's when our healing process begins. Whether you are here in your physical body or on the other side without your physical body, you will still need to address that inner pain.

People get angry when I tell them about Limbo, because for so many people the prospect of suicide seems like a real option for pain relief. But clearly, this is not so! One way or another, we still have to face our inner pain and do whatever is necessary to heal it.

For those of you who have a loved one who has committed suicide, there is something you can do for that soul. Visualize them and tell them to look for the help that is available to them. Tell them to look for the white light of heaven and go towards it. Tell them they do not need to stay stuck where they are. Say it once or twice a day. Yes, you can say it out loud. They can hear you. After awhile, you will sense a release, and this is an indication that they have moved on. The sense of release is very slight, so don't get caught up in whether or not they have gone on. Simply say it until it no longer feels necessary.

Meanwhile, be assured that you can heal from whatever pain you are in. But you cannot do it by yourself. Please, if you are thinking that suicide is a solution, reach out to as many people as you can. Someone will help you!

SECTION III

From Author to Reader

Huckleberry Finn

Work consists of whatever a body is obliged *to do . . .*
Play consists of whatever a body is not obliged to do.
—Mark Twain

I was thinking that I had completed this book, but something just didn't feel like it was quite finished. I could not figure out what area I had forgotten to write about. So I put a crayon in my nondominant hand and asked my inner child what area was missing. She wrote out "HUCKLEBERRY FINN." What? I asked. I could not figure out what that meant, so I asked her to tell me. She wrote "FUN" in big letters!

"Oh," I said, "you want me to write a chapter on fun?"

She replied, "FUN THINGS TO DO."

I thought about this. It sure felt like the missing piece.

Being a person who, for a long time, hasn't been comfortable having fun, I asked others what they do for fun. See the following list of suggestions for you to think about, just in case you sometimes get stuck not knowing what to do for fun.

go to an amusement park
watch TV
read
hang out with friends
rent a movie
make a movie
go roller skating
go for a drive
take pictures
go shopping
sew
go to the zoo
go out to dinner
make jewelry
eat ice cream
get a new hairdo
draw pictures
go roller-blading
go to the movies
cook/bake
go swimming
play board games
go jogging
go for a walk

go to sporting events
play tennis
plan a party
join a club
wash your car
make T-shirts
work out at a health club
hot tub
ride your bike
go dancing
go boating
go motorcycling
go fishing
go ice skating
go bowling
do yard work
go skiing
take dance lessons
grocery shop
get a massage
fly a kite
gourmet cooking
go on a picnic
go hunting
buy yourself a toy
that you always wanted
knit
crochet
go hang gliding
arrange flowers
go to a museum
embroider
see a play in a theater
make a model
collect things
do volunteer work
do jigsaw puzzles
grow a garden
play an instrument
go on vacation
go to a concert
go to the races
go camping
clean your house
buy silly cards for friends
get a manicure or pedicure
mow the lawn
swing on a swing
slide down a slide
cross-country skiing
downhill skiing
sports
write poetry
go to the lake
go out to eat
go horseback riding
meditate
visit shut-ins
throw a party/entertain
pick apples
go to art festivals
go for a plane ride
collect stamps

Last, but not least, I wanted to include in this chapter my own variation of the principles that Robert Fulghum presented in his book *All I Ever Needed To Know I Learned in Kindergarten.* Here's my own simplified short list—just for fun:

1. Share everything.
2. Always play fair.
3. Don't hurt anybody—including yourself.
4. Put things back where you found them.
5. Clean up after yourself.
6. Never take anything that isn't yours.
7. If you hurt somebody, tell them you're sorry.
8. Take care of your body—with plenty of love.
9. Give yourself little treats from time to time, to remind you of how much you appreciate being you.
10. Make it a goal to create balance and harmony in your life.
11. Every day of your life, try to learn something new, think some, play some, do something creative and fun.
12. Be still and talk with your inner child each day.
13. You are never alone. There are always those around you who can help, whether a friend, family member, professional person, or your Higher Power. Help is always as close as a thought.
14. Each day, be open to the mysteries of life, the wonder and awe of it all.
15. Each day, take a moment to think about the growth of life in its many forms, from the tiniest plant to the largest animal—and how we are a part of that.
16. All things that live—flowers, kittens, trees, even ourselves—must someday die. And this, too, is part of the mystery and awe of the world.
17. Each day, put aside some time to turn to the Higher Power and ask for guidance, willing to look and listen as a complete beginner.

Recommended Reading

If you get too many things going at once, you won't know what to do or who to listen to.
—Anonymous

After I had had about two years of sobriety, I asked my AA sponsor (someone who acts like a big brother or sister and who teaches his or her "sponsees" the ropes of the program and about sobriety), if I could go to therapy. He asked me to recite the twelve steps to him. I couldn't. He told me to stick to one thing until I knew what I was doing, before I went on to the next thing. He said that it was important to keep it simple. He said, "If you get too many things going on at once, you won't know what to do or who to listen to." I have never forgotten those words. They have helped me immensely over the years.

I was recently in the home of a female client. This woman has a bad back. She had an enormous library of books on health, nutrition, exercise, spirituality, several well-known self-help books, and New Age books. At first, I felt a little intimidated because I assumed that if she read all of those books and lived by them, there wouldn't be much that I could offer her besides healings. . . . It was quite the contrary. She was very anxious and uptight. She had no sense of peacefulness. She was very controlling about the healing sessions. She wanted them to be done "just so."

After I had channeled only a couple of healings for her, she was very disappointed that she hadn't been healed. Her back still hurt. I asked her if she had read the books in her library. Yes, she had read them, hadn't everyone? I asked her if she had done any of the things suggested in Louise Hay's book, *You Can Heal Your Life.* She told me that she didn't have the time. She said that she was meaning to get to the exercises in the various books, but because of work or whatever, she just never found the time.

She was very impatient with the healings. Everyday after our session, I could feel her disappointment that her back was still painful. She had given me one week to heal her back. At the end of that week, she told me she no longer wanted to try healings, that she was going to try something else. John had made some suggestions to her through a psychic reading about some issues that she had stored in her back, but she said that she just didn't have time to "mess around" with feelings and therapy. It was such an odd feeling that day when I left her house. I didn't know what it was until I experienced it again with another client.

This man had cancer. He was willing to spend all the money he had to get healed, but he didn't feel that he should have to make any internal changes in himself. He, too, had an enormous library of self-help, New Age, nutritional, exercise, spiritual, psychic, and astrological books. He had read all of them. John told him in a reading that he needed to find a spiritual teacher and to get going on a spiritual path. He needed to get out of his head and start clearing out those negative beliefs. John said that this man believed that if he just had all of the knowledge about his body and his disease that he could possibly learn, that he then would be in control of his health. Then the cancer would go away.

John talked a lot about the other areas of this man's life that needed some attention, such as the emotional and spiritual issues in his soul and body. The man reassured me several times that he would look at the emotional issues that came up in a psychic reading. He would start looking for a teacher who could guide him onto a spiritual path. Yet, every time that I asked him what he was doing, he would show me a new stack of books or a new-fangled machine that he had just purchased to get rid of the cancer. He went from one thing to the next, but I never saw any change. This was the same thing that had happened to the client with a bad back. After a very short time of doing healings, he told me that he was going to try something else.

In both situations, I felt bad that more time wasn't allowed for the healing energy to work, but at the same time, it seemed as if I was banging my head against the wall. Both people were very impatient. They wanted immediate results. They weren't willing to do any emotional or spiritual work for themselves. A friend of mine said, "It sounds like they thought of you as just one more book, a quick fix which didn't work, so on to the next thing." That sure seemed to fit with how I was feeling!

I share these two stories with you because it's important to me to suggest that you don't run out and buy all of the "in" books. First, you need to be patient with your healing process. Second, when you do shop for books, shop with your intuition. Don't buy a book because the cover looks good or because everyone else is reading it. It may not fit your needs. Perhaps you're not ready for it yet. If you have a friend who has been on a spiritual journey for quite some time and you're just starting, the books that he or she reads might not fit your needs. Third, when you do purchase some books, please take each one slowly, taking from each one as much as you can.

When I first read *Living in the Light* by Shakti Gawain and *You Can Heal Your Life* by Louise Hay, I spent a lot of time with each book. As my sponsor said, "If you get too many things going at once, you won't know what to do or who to listen to." So I guess what this is all about is:

Take your time. Enjoy each book. Take everything from the book that it has to offer.

There is no contest. We are not in a hurry. Enjoy this wonderful healing process.

My frustration in preparing the book list included here as Appendix B is that I don't want you to be limited by my suggestions. There are so many wonderful books on the market. My fear is that I'm forgetting half of the books that probably belong on this list. Please follow your intuition when buying a book. Get what "feels right," and you won't go wrong!

Epilogue

So here we are at the end. It feels sad to be saying good-bye to you. It sure feels as if we've travelled down a long road together.

I also feel very excited for you! Once you get rid of all that old garbage, you are finally going to know how special you are. You're breaking old patterns. Your future will not be full of pain and self-doubt. You're reaching for freedom. You "deserve"—remember back in Chapter 18 when we worked this one through?—every ounce of happiness that you will experience!

Carlos, a wonderful psychic friend, used to tell me to turn my scars to stars. I believe that's what I have done. By removing the pain from your memories, by healing those negative beliefs about yourself, and looking for the good in the pain that you've endured, you too are turning your scars into stars.

We don't have to wait to get back to the Garden of Eden. It's here. Right now. We've missed it because it's inside of us. And until now we've been looking outside. When we get free from the old stuck patterns, we've arrived. We're home. It's the *it* that we've all been seeking. It's time to know that you are the most important person in your world. We will not have world peace until we all heal ourselves *first*. Remember what Jesus said: "Love thy neighbor as thyself." No more excuses. No more delays. It's time to go for it!

God Bless You On Your Journey!

Appendices

APPENDIX A

List of Health Care Alternatives

This list is adapted from Kristin Gottschalk Olsen's book, *The Encyclopedia of Alternative Health Care,* published by Pocket Books in New York, 1989.

Acupressure

Many different massage techniques can be grouped under this umbrella term. Basically, those massage techniques that are termed acupressure stimulate various body energy points with the use of pressure. Usually the energy points to which the pressure is applied are those recognized by acupuncture. The application of pressure is a means of stimulating the body's internal healing energies. There are five major types of acupressure: Acu-Yoga, Do-In, Jin Shin, Shiatsu, and Tui Na.

Acu-Yoga. Different yoga postures are used that involve the entire body. These exercises will energize the acupressure points.

Do-In. In this massage technique, which includes a variety of exercises using body movement, one self-administers his or her own acupressure.

Jin Shin. This is a gentle technique in which pressure is applied to selected points for one to five minutes at a time. Patients are treated while they are in meditation.

Shiatsu. This is a series of tapping or stretching, rhythmic finger pressure techniques. These are applied along the body's energy meridians for a very brief period.

Tui Na. Different hand motions are used in this Chinese method to stimulate the various acupressure points.

Acupuncture

This treatment is an integral part of Chinese medicine, often referred to as Traditional Chinese Medicine. Selected acupuncture points on the surface of the skin play a role in the functioning of every body part. Tiny needles are placed in selected acupuncture points that need stimulation. In addition, heat or pressure (acupressure or massage) can also be applied.

Alexander Technique

Frederick M. Alexander, an Austrian actor, developed this technique whereby the body or mind could reduce any tension by overcoming improper body movements or posture. Several lessons are presented under the guidance of an Alexander teacher that explore how one can regain the body's natural balances that have been lost in stressful situations.

Applied Kinesiology

This is a technique using "muscle testing" for neurological disorders. Based on classical Chinese acupuncture, applied kinesiology relates the use of neurovascular and neurolymphatic reflexes to the body's chemical, mental, and structural regulation mechanisms. Chiropractors often use applied kinesiology to correct muscle spasms.

Aromatherapy

This technique uses extracts from cultivated or wild species of plants for various therapies (classic herbal medicine or beauty). The plant extracts contain specific compounds that produce various effects on the body. These extracts may be prescribed by physicians for internal use or are more frequently administered with massage, steam inhalation, salves and ointments, or bathing. A variety of illnesses have been treated with aromatherapy: acne, anxiety, circulatory problems, depression, obesity, ruptured capillaries, rheumatism, and stress. It is advisable to use these extracts only under the advice of an aromatherapist, since many of the extracted oils can be poisonous in larger quantities.

Autogenic Training & Therapy

Dr. Johannes Schultz, a Berlin psychiatrist, and several of his students formulated the exercises that became known as Autogenic Therapy. This technique uses different exercises to focus the patient's attention on creating a state of relaxation for the mind and body. It is a type of self-hypnosis that induces experiences similar to, but not actually, the hypnotic state. By generating a state of deep relaxation, one can tap into the self-regenerative powers of the body.

Ayurveda

Ayurveda, meaning the knowledge of life, is an ancient medical practice from India. It incorporates many different concepts into a practical life science for everyday living. A patient is initially evaluated by an Ayurvedic physician for body type and current body condition. From this, a patient is given a picture of his/her general state of health in terms of the three bioforces: kapha, pitta, and vata. After this session, the Ayurvedic consulting begins: a series of living styles, treatments, and therapies are prescribed.

Bach Flower Remedies or Flower Essences

These flower extracts were created when it was discovered that local vegetation contained essential healing powers. A flower essence is created by exposing flowers immersed in water to sunlight. This process infuses the water with the flower's particular life energies and elements. Initially, Edward Bach created 38 flower remedies. Richard Katz has also added 72 flower essences, using plants native to California. The principle of Bach flower remedies is that plants possess energetic properties that are able to reconnect body and soul.

Bioenergetics

Bioenergetics or body-oriented psychotherapies incorporate the healing power of touching. Touch has been used since ancient times as a means of healing. These can range from a therapist applying pressure to a patient to a more nurturing method of holding the client. Many of the psychotherapeutic techniques were developed from findings of Dr. Georg Groddeck and Dr. Wilhelm Reich.

Biofeedback Training

In this technique, the patient learns to listen to and control the various body functions with information provided from various machines. Unconscious physiological functions become known with the use of these machines.

Chiropractic

Chiropractors, working with their hands, use various manipulating massage techniques to adjust the spinal column. While classic chiropractic treatment is limited to spinal adjustments, more liberal practitioners include any health care method except drugs or surgery. Chiropractic is useful for pains or disorders that have not yet developed into a more serious disease condition.

Colon Hydrotherapy

Colon hydrotherapy or colonics is a technique to gently flush out the intestines. Normal enemas only cleanse the descending colon and rectum.

Feldenkrais Method

In this method, the patient learns to use movement as a means of creating a sense of newness. Feldenkrais can be taught in group (awareness through movement) or private (functional integration) sessions. Patients focus on the ease of movement and how their bodies are being misused. The heightened awareness allows one to develop the means of healthy body movements.

Healers

There are many different kinds of healers, all of whom use powers developed through the use of intuition or lengthy apprenticeships. Energy, in some form or another, is channeled to the patient using various techniques. Healers use many different techniques for healing: absentee healing, clairvoyance, energies, faith, magnetic energy, laying-on of hands, psychic abilities, and spirituality.

Herbal Medicine

Herbal medicine is useful for eliminating specific illnesses. It is present in virtually every culture, forming an important component of healing ceremonies and remedies passed from generation to generation. Shamans and medicine men/women use many different herbal remedies to treat disease. Any plant parts, whether leaves, stems, flowers, seeds, roots, or underground storage organs, can be used in herbal remedies. The plant extracts are formulated into various types of remedies including tinctures, ointments, salves, lotions, liniments, or oils; teas; decoctions (the herbs are concentrated by boiling and straining); mastication aids (the chewing of plant parts); extract drops that are applied orally; enemas or douches; suppositories to draw out toxins; essences added to baths; steam inhalation; syrups and poultices.

Homeopathy

Homeopathy, which means to use a similar sickness, is based on the thought that causal agents that create illness can be used as cures when they are applied in extremely minute quantities. Homeopathic remedies are made of natural substances from animals, plants, and chemicals.

Hypnosis

Hypnosis is a technique where patients are induced into an altered state of consciousness, somewhere between sleeping and being fully awake. Patients receive thoughts or ideas from the hypnotist in a therapeutic setting. Hypnotic states are similar to those that each of us has experienced: daydreaming or becoming mesmerized by monotonous situations. Hypnosis is a very useful therapeutic tool and can be used to remove unhealthful living habits.

Iridology

This technique is a modified form of reflexology where the conditions of the body are "reflected" in the eyes. The iris of the eye is examined for various body disorders, providing a complete picture of the patient's psychological, emotional, and physiological condition. Iridologists rely on the use of eye maps to understand the specific body conditions.

Martial Arts

There are many different forms of martial arts, originating in the Orient and South America, that are useful techniques in self-defense, expression via body movement, and understanding of oneself. These techniques arose from combat or ritualistic dancing and include Aikido (Japanese), Chi Gung or Qi Gong (Chinese), Judo (Japanese), Jujitsu (Japanese), Karate (Japanese), Kendo (Japanese), Kung Fu (Chinese), Tae Kwon Do (Korean), or T'ai Chi Ch'uan (Chinese).

Massage

In this technique, the patient's body is systematically stroked, kneaded, or massaged to relieve various disorders. Usually masseuses and masseurs use massage oils to reduce the friction of body contact. Since everyone responds to touch, massage is a very sensuous healing technique. Many different massage techniques are available.

Myotherapy

This technique was created by Bonnie Prudden to defuse muscle trigger points (irritable muscle points that can cause substantial pain). Myotherapists apply pressure to the trigger points, as well as providing exercises to retrain the muscles.

Naturopathic Medicine

Naturopathy combines various healing methods with natural therapeutics into a healing system of nature. It is a drugless therapy, using the curing abilities of the elements (sun, water, air, and earth). As with many other techniques, symptoms in the body are regarded as a means whereby the body begins to heal itself. Naturopathic professionals may also use X-rays, laboratory tests, obstetrics, etc. in the treatment process.

Nutrition Therapy

Food or our diet provide more than nourishment for the body. They also are important tools for preventative health care. Beyond the many different types of diet books that are available, nutrition therapy may also be used to treat eating disorders.

Osteopathy

Osteopathy was developed prior to chiropractic and focuses on maintaining the body's structural balance to allow healing. Osteopaths are medically trained as physicians and can prescribe drugs or herbs in the treatment of diseases.

Past Life Therapy

In this technique, information from past lifetimes is obtained from either hypnosis of the client or psychic abilities of the therapist. Various traumatic life situations are looked for that may be causing illnesses or disorders in the present lifetime. These situations are examined to enable the client to learn the lesson(s) from these past traumas. This treatment differs from past life regression, where past lifetime information is gathered but not used in a therapeutic sense with the patient.

Polarity Therapy

This therapeutic technique was developed by Dr. Randolph Stone. He based it primarily on East Indian principles of Ayurveda. It is designed to create an energy balance within the body through the use of nutrition therapy, exercises, touch therapy, and emotional or mental balancing. A polarity therapist works primarily by placing his/her hands on the patient's energy system centers to direct the energy flow in the proper directions throughout the body.

Reflexology

Reflexology traces back to ancient Chinese medicine. Hand strokes or the application of pressure to a body part is used for relaxation of muscles or to stimulate the body's healing system. In hand or foot reflexology, two of the classic forms, a map of the body is seen on a patient's palm or sole of the feet. Applying reflexology to specific areas of the map will stimulate specific areas of the body.

Reiki Healing

This healing system is derived from Tibetan masters. In Reiki healing sessions, practitioners channel a Universal Life Energy force to clients or their family members. The energy is transmitted by lightly touching the hands on specific body parts. It is useful to balance any of the four bodies (mental, emotional, physical, or spiritual).

Rolfing

Rolfing or structural integration consists of ten sessions of bodywork where the connective tissues are manipulated. The goal is to create an aligned body that can efficiently use its energy. In rolfing, the muscle length is increased, allowing for the attainment of optimal body posture.

Rosen Method Bodywork

This uses talking and touch to create a state of muscle relaxation. Patients learn how to use their breath as a means of enhancing flexibility in the body structure. The body is believed to be a storehouse of events, memories, emotions, or traumas that provide useful clues in how the patient lives life. Each of the uncovered issues are dealt with in a therapeutic setting, thus encouraging the healing process.

Shamanism

This is a spiritual and medicinal practice that exists in all cultures in the world. Illness is viewed as a disharmony, either in individuals, families, or entire tribes. Shamans use many different means, by which an altered consciousness state is attained, to communicate in realms other than reality. These altered consciousness states are necessary in order for the patient to find connections with nature or the spirits.

Therapeutic Touch

This technique was recently developed in the medical profession for nurses and other health care professionals to enhance patient treatment and recovery. It is fundamentally based on the concept of psychic healing, the transfer of energy from one human to another.

Trager Approach

When in a relaxed state (termed "hook up"), patients are submitted to a combination of mind movement techniques and "hands-on" treatments. These are used to break up living patterns or styles that have served to decrease muscle action.

Yoga

This Indian practice is a means of deliverance from body disorders by controlling whatever may be causing the disruption of peace and harmony. Mind control is used to eliminate the powerful ego and actions of the intellect. The goal in Yoga is to obtain the ultimate integration of the spiritual, mental, emotional, and physical bodies. Yoga exercises involve different body positioning and movements, dietary disciplines, and breathing exercises.

APPENDIX B

Recommended Reading List

Addictions

Becnel, Barbara Cottman. *Parents Who Help Their Children Overcome Drugs.* Los Angeles: Lowell House, 1989.

Casey, Karen. *If Only I Could Quit/Recovering from Nicotine Addiction.* New York: Harper/Hazelden, 1987.

Nakken, Craig. *The Addictive Personality.* San Francisco: Harper & Row, 1988.

Peele, Stanton. *Love and Addiction.* New York: Taplinger Publishing Co., 1975.

Peluso, Emanuel and Lucy Silvay Peluso. *Women & Drugs.* Rockville, MD: U.S. Dept. of Health and Human Services, Public Health Service, Alcohol, Drug Abuse and Mental Health Administration, National Institution on Drug Abuse; Washington, D.C. For sale by the Supt. of Docs., U.S. G.P.O., 1983.

Adult Children of Alcoholics

Ackerman, Robert. *Perfect Daughters/Adult Daughters of Alcoholics.* Deerfield, FL: Health Communications, 1989.

Black, Claudia. *It Will Never Happen To Me!* Denver: MAC Printing & Publication Division.

Carnes, Patrick. *A Gentle Path Through the Twelve Steps.* Minneapolis: CompCare, 1989.

Friel, John and Linda Friel. *Adult Children—The Secrets of Dysfunctional Families.* Deerfield, FL: Health Communications, 1990.

Friel, John and Linda Friel. *An Adult Child's Guide to What's Normal.* Deerfield, FL: Health Communications, 1990.

Larsen, Earnie. *Adult Children of Dysfunctional Families.* Brooklyn Park, MN: E. Larsen Enterprises, 1984.

Lerner, Rokclle. *Daily Affirmations for Adult Children of Alcoholics.* Deerfield, FL: Health Communications, 1985.

Wegscheider-Cruse, Sharon. *The Miracle of Recovery.* Deerfield, FL: Health Communications, 1989.

Woititz, Janet Geringer. *Adult Children of Alcoholics.* Hollywood, FL: Health Communications, 1983.

Woititz, Janet Geringer. *Struggle for Intimacy.* Pompano Beach, FL: Health Communications, 1985.

Woititz, Janet Geringer and Alan Garner. *Lifeskills For Adult Chilren.* Deerfield, FL: Health Communications, 1990.

Assertiveness

Alberti. *Your Perfect Right.* San Luis Obispo, CA: Impact Publishers, 1986.

Cancer Therapy

Simonton, Simonton, and Creighton. *Getting Well Again.* New York: Bantam Books, 1978.

Codependency

Beattie, Melody. *Codependent No More.* New York: Harper & Row, 1987.

Beattie, Melody. *Beyond Codependency and Getting Better All The Time.* New York: Harper & Row, 1989.

Beattie, Melody. *The Language of Letting Go.* New York: HarperCollins, 1990.

Cermak, Timmen. *A Time To Heal.* Los Angeles: J.P. Tarcher; New York: Distributed by St. Martin's Press, 1988.

Kellogg, Terry. *Broken Toys, Broken Dreams.* (Also any of Terry's tapes.) Deerfield, FL: Health Communications, 1989.

Mellody, Pia. *Facing Codependence.* San Francisco: Harper & Row, 1989.

Ricketson, Susan Cooley. *The Dilemma of Love.* Deerfield, FL: Health Communications, 1989.

Wegscheider-Cruse, Sharon. *Choicemaking.* Pompano Beach, FL: Health Communications, 1985.

Depression

Burns, David D. *Feeling Good—The New Mood Therapy.* New York: Morrow, 1980.

Greist, John H. and James W. Jefferson. *Depression and Its Treatment.* New York: Warner Books, 1984.

Healing

Brennan, Barbara Ann. *Hands of Light. A Guide to Healing Through the Human Energy Field.* Toronto and New York: Bantam Books, 1987.

Burns, Echo Bodine. *Hands That Heal.* San Diego: ACS Publishing, 1985.

Siegel, Bernie. *Love, Medicine, & Miracles.* New York: Harper & Row, 1986.

Siegel, Bernie. *Peace, Love, & Healing.* New York: Harper & Row, 1989.

Huckleberry Finn

The humor section of any bookstore.

Inner Child

Cappachione, Lucia. *Recovery of Your Inner Child.* New York: Simon & Schuster, 1991.

Whitfield, Charles. *A Gift to Myself.* Deerfield, FL: Health Communications, 1990.

Whitfield, Charles. *Healing The Child Within.* Deerfield, FL: Health Communications, 1987.

Inspirational

Kopp, Sheldon. *If You Meet Buddha On The Road, Kill Him.* Ben Lomond, CA: Science and Behavior Books, 1972.

Lazaris. *Lazaris—The Sacred Journey; You and Your Higher Self.* Synergy Publishing, 1987.

Rodegast, Pat and Judith Stanton (eds.). *Emmanuel's Book.* New York: Bantam Books, 1985.

Rodegast, Pat and Judith Stanton (eds.). *Emmanuel's Book II.* New York: Bantam Books, 1989.

Siegel, Bernie. *Love, Medicine, and Miracles.* New York: Harper & Row, 1986.

Siegel, Bernie. *Peace, Love, and Healing.* New York: Harper & Row, 1989.

Intuition

Gawain, Shakti. *Living In The Light.* Mill Valley, CA: Nataraj Publishing, 1986.

Loss and Grief

Colgrove, Melba. *How To Survive The Loss of a Loved One.* New York: Lion Press, 1976.

Meditation

Beattie, Melody. *Language of Letting Go—Daily Meditations.* New York: HarperCollins, 1990.

Each Day A New Beginning. New York: HarperCollins, 1990.

Hazelden Meditation Series. Many different meditation books.

Men

Abbott, Franklin (ed.). *New Men, New Minds.* Freedom, CA: Crossing Press, 1987.

Farrell, Warren. *Why Men Are The Way They Are.* New York: McGraw-Hill, 1986.

Fossum, Merle. *Catching Fire.* New York: Harper & Row, 1989.

Goldberg, Herb. *The Hazards of Being Male.* New York: New American Library, 1977.

Goldberg, Herb. *The New Male.* New York: Morrow, 1979.

Hazelden Meditation Series. *Touchstones/Daily Meditations for Men.* New York: HarperCollins, 1986.

Johnson, Robert. *He.* King of Prussia, PA: Religions Publishing Co., 1974.

Lee, John. *The Flying Boy/Healing the Wounded Man.* New York: Crown Books, 1987.

Levinson, Daniel. *The Seasons of a Man's Life.* New York: Knopf, 1978.

McGill, Michael. *The McGill Report on Male Intimacy.* New York: Holt, Rinehart & Winston, 1985.

Miller, Stuart. *Men & Friendship.* Boston: Houghton Mifflin, 1983.

Naifeh, Steven and Gregory White Smith. *Why Can't Men Open Up?* New York: C.N. Potter, 1984.

Nelson, James. *The Intimate Connection.* New York: Morrow, 1985.

Pleck, Joseph and Jack Sawyer (eds.). *Men and Masculinity.* Englewood Cliffs, NJ: Prentice-Hall, 1974.

Menopause

Gray, Madeline. *The Changing Years.* New York: Doubleday & Co., Inc., 1951.

New Age

McLaine, Shirley. *Out On A Limb.* New York: Bantam Books, 1983.

Pill Addiction

Gordon, Barbara. *I'm Dancing As Fast As I Can.* New York: Harper & Row, 1979.

Reincarnation

Bach, Richard. *One.* New York: Silver Arrow Books, 1988.

Bach, Richard. *Bridge Across Forever.* New York: Morrow, 1984.

Montgomery, Ruth. *The World Beyond.* New York: Coward, McCann & Geoghegan, 1971.

Moody, Raymond. *Life After Life.* Boston: G.K. Hall, 1977.

Self-Help

Alcoholics Anonymous World Services. *Alcoholics Anonymous.* New York: Alcoholics Anonymous World Service, 1976.

Bradshaw, John. *Homecoming.* New York: Bantam Books, 1990.

Bradshaw, John. *Healing the Shame That Binds You.* Pompano Beach, FL: Health Communications, 1989.

Bradshaw, John. *Bradshaw: On The Family. A Revolutionary Way of Self-Discovery.* Deerfield, FL: Health Communications, 1988.

Chopich and Paul. *Healing Your Aloneness.* San Francisco: Harper & Row, 1990.

Gawain, Shakti. *Living in the Light.* Mill Valley, CA: Nataraj Publishing, 1986.

Gorski, Terence. *Passages Through Recovery.* San Francisco: Harper & Row, 1989.

Hay, Louise. *You Can Heal Your Life.* Farmingdale, NY: Coleman Publishing, 1984.

Hay, Louise. *Heal Your Body.* Santa Monica, CA: Hay House, 1982.

Larsen, Earnest. *Building Healthy Adult Relationships.* Brooklyn Park, MN: E. Larsen Enterprises, 1988.

Larsen, Earnie. All of his books! He also has tapes and workshops available.

Lerner, Harriet. *The Dance of Anger: Woman's Guide to Changing the Patterns of Intimate Relationships.* New York: Harper & Row, 1989.

Lerner, Harriet. *The Dance of Intimacy: A Woman's Guide to Courageous Acts of Change in Key Relationships.* New York: Harper & Row, 1989.

Norwood, Robin. *Women Who Love Too Much.* Los Angeles: J.P. Tarcher, 1985.

Paul, Jordan and Margaret Paul. *Do I Have to Give Up Me to be Loved by You?* Minneapolis: CompCare Publications, 1983.

Peck, M. Scott. *The Road Less Travelled.* New York: Simon & Schuster, 1978.

Powell, John. *Why Am I Afraid to Tell You Who I Am?* Allen, TX: Tabor Publications, 1969.

Powell, John. *Why Am I Afraid to Love?* Chicago: Argus Communications, 1967.

Rosellini, Gayle and Mark Worden. *Of Course You're Angry.* San Francisco: Harper & Row, 1985.

Rubin. *The Angry Book.* New York: Collier Books, 1970.

Schaef, Ann Wilson. *Escape From Intimacy.* San Francisco: Harper & Row, 1989.

Schaef, Ann Wilson. *Women's Reality.* Minneapolis: Winston Press, 1981.

Sheehy, Gail. *Passages: Predictable Crisis of Adult Life.* New York: Dutton, 1976.

Sheehy, Gail. *Pathfinders. Overcoming the Crisis of Adult Life and Finding Your Own Path to Well Being.* New York: Bantam Books, 1981.

Steadman, Alice. *Who's The Matter With Me?* Marina Del Ray, CA: DeVorss, 1966.

Woititz, Janet Geringer. *Struggle for Intimacy.* Pompano Beach, FL: Health Communications, 1985.

Sex Addiction

Hope and Recovery: A Twelve Step Guide for Healing from Compulsive Sexual Behavior. Minneapolis: CompCare, 1987.

Carnes, Patrick. *Out of the Shadows: Understanding Sexual Addiction.* Minneapolis: CompCare, 1987.

Davis Kasl, Charlotte. *Women, Sex, and Addiction.* New York: ticknor & Fields, 1989.

Hunter, Mic. *The First Step for People In Relationships With Sex Addicts.* Minneapolis, CompCare, 1989.

Schneider, Jennifer. *Back From Betrayal.* San Francisco: Harper & Row, 1988.

Sexual Abuse

Bass, Ellen and Laura Davis. *The Courage To Heal—A Guide for Women Survivors of Child Abuse.* New York: Harper & Row, 1985.

Davis, Laura. *The Courage To Heal Workbook.* New York: Harper & Row, 1990.

Davis, Laura. *Allies In Healing.* New York: Harper Perennial, 1991.

Lew, Mike. *Victims No More—Men Recovering From Incest and Other Sexual-Child Abuse.* New York: Nevraumont Publishing Co., 1988.

Mautz, Wendy. *Sexual Healing Journey.* New York: HarperCollins Publishing, 1991.

Utain, Marsha and Barbara Oliver. *Scream Louder: Through Hell and Healing With An Incest Survivor and Her Therapist.* Deerfield, FL: Health Communications, 1989.

Shame

Bradshaw, John. *Healing the Shame That Binds You.* Pompano Beach, FL: Health Communications, 1989.

Fossum and Mason. *Facing Shame: Families in Recovery.* New York: Norton & Co., Inc., 1986.

Hazelton, Deborah M. *The Courage to See/Daily Affirmations.* Center City, MN: Hazelden Foundation.

Monahan, Ray. *Self Esteem Subliminal Audio Tape.* Cener City, MN: Hazelden, 1989.

Spirituality

Cady, Emilie. *Lessons In Truth.* Kansas City: Unity School of Christianity, 1946.

Fox, Emmet. *Sermon On The Mount.* New York: Harper & Row, 1938.

Gawain, Shakti. *Creative Visualization.* San Rafael, CA: New World Library, 1978, and New York: Bantam Books, 1993.

Keyes, Ken. *Handbook to Higher Consciousness.* Coos Bay, OR: Love Line Books, 1975.

Mandino, Og. *The Greatest Salesman in the World.* New York: F. Fell, 1968.

Mary. *You are God.* DeVorss.

Peale, Norman Vincent. *The Power of Positive Thinking.* Englewood Cliffs, NJ: Prentice-hall, 1956.

Peck, M. Scott. *The Road Less Travelled;* also *A New Psychology of Love: Traditional Values and Spiritual Growth.* New York: Simon & Schuster, 1978.

Prather, Hugh. *Notes to Myself.* Lafayette, CA: Real People Press, 1970.

Stress

Freudenberger, Herbert. *Burn Out.* Garden City, NY: Anchor Press, 1980.

Weight

Gordon-Stoltz. *The Food Fix: A Recovery Guide for Destructive Eaters.* Englewood Cliffs, NJ: Prentice-Hall, 1983.

Hazelden Meditation Series. *Food For Thought/Daily Meditations for Overeaters.* Center City, MN: Hazelden Foundation, 1980.

Hollis, Judy. *Fat Is A Family Affair.* New York: Hazelden, Harper, 1985.

McFarland, Barbara and Anne Marie Erb. *Abstinence in Action.* San Francisco, Harper & Row, 1988.

McFarland, Barbara and Tyeis Baker-Bauman. *Shame and Body Image.* Deerfield, FL: Health Communications, 1990.

Orbach, Susie. *Fat Is a Feminist Issue. I & II.* New York: Berkeley Books, 1987 (II); and New York: Paddington Press, 1978 (regular).

Wellness

Boston Women's Health. *Our Bodies, Ourselves.* New York: Simon & Schuster, 1976.

Gottschalk Olsen, Kristin. *The Encyclopedia of Alternative Health Care.* New York: Pocket Books, 1989.

Wood, Matthew. *Seven Herbs: Plants as Teachers.* Berkeley, CA: North Atlantic Books, 1986.

Quotations Used in *Passion to Heal*

Chapter 4

John Bradshaw. "The Child Within." *New Realities*. July/August, 1990. pp. 11-15, 36-42.

Chapter 5

John and Linda Friel. *Adult Children—The Secrets of Dysfunctional Families*. Deerfield, FL: Health Communications, 1990. pp. 18-22, 53-56.

Chapter 7

Overeaters Anonymous, *A Disease of the Body*, p. 90. Torrance: CA: Overeaters Anonymous, Inc., 1980.

Sexual Addicts Anonymous. *The Twenty Questions of Sexual Addicts Anonymous*.

Chapter 8

Bernie Siegel. *New Age Journal*, May-June, 1989. p. 37.

Barry Weinhold and Janae Weinhold. *Breaking Free of the Copendency Trap*. Walpole, NH: Stillpoint Publishing, 1989. pp. 8-9.

Chapter 11

Herb Goldberg. *The Hazards of Being Male* ("Impossible Binds" chapter). New York, NY: Sanford J. Greenburger Associates, Inc., 1976. pp. i, 86.

Jach Pursel. "Lazaris," *Body, Mind, and Spirit*. October, 1989.

Sidney Jourard. *The Transparent Self*. Princeton, NJ: Van Nostrand Co., 1971. p. 40.

Chapter 12

Shakti Gawain. *Living in the Light*. Mill Valley, CA: Nataraj Publishing (originally published by New World Library, 1986).

Chapter 14

Golden Valley Health Center, "Anorexia—Early Signs and Symptoms." Golden Valley, MN: Golden Valley Health Center.

Golden Valley Health Center, "Bulimia—Early Signs and Symptoms." Golden Valley, MN: golden Valley Health Center.

Chapter 16

Emmanuel. *Emmanuel's Book.* New York: Bantam Books, Inc., 1985. pp. 18-19.

Alcoholics Anonymous. *Alcoholics Anonymous*, "The Eighth and Ninth Steps of AA." New York: Alcoholics Anonymous World Services, 1955. pp. 59-80.

Chapter 17

Herbert J. Freudenberger. *Burn Out.* New York: Bantam Books, Inc., 1980. pp. 18-19.

Alcoholics Anonymous. *Alcoholics Anonymous*, "The Tenth Step of AA." New York: Alcoholics Anonymous World Services, 1955. p. 60.

John H. Griest and James W. Jefferson. *Depression and Its Treatment.* Washington, D.C.: American Psychiatric Press, 1992. pp. 4-8.

John H. Griest and James W. Jefferson. "Beck Depression Inventory (BDI)," *Depression and Its Treatment.* New York: Warner Books, by arrangement with American Psychiatric Press, Inc., Washington, D.C., 1985. pp. 22-26.

To receive more information
on Echo Bodine and her work,
write to:

Echo Bodine
P.O. Box 19065
Minneapolis, MN 55419

Nataraj Publishing

is committed to acting as a catalyst for change and transformation in the world by providing books and tapes on the leading edge in the fields of personal and social consciousness growth. "Nataraj" is a Sanskrit word referring to the creative, transformative power of the universe. For more information on our company, please contact us at:

Nataraj Publishing
1561 So. Novato Blvd., Suite A
Novato, CA 94947
Phone: (415) 899-9666
Fax: (415) 899-9667

Other Books and Tapes from Nataraj Publishing

Books

Living in the Light: A Guide to Personal and Planetary Transformation. By Shakti Gawain with Laurel King. The recognized classic on developing intuition and using it as a guide in living your life. (Trade paperback $9.95)

Living in the Light Workbook. By Shakti Gawain. Following up her bestseller, *Living in the Light.* Shakti has created a workbook to help us apply these principles to our lives in very practical ways. (Trade paperback $12.95)

Return to the Garden: A Journey of Discovery. By Shakti Gawain. Shakti reveals her path to self-discovery and personal power and shows us how to return to our personal garden and live on earth in a natural and balanced way. (Trade paperback $9.95)

Awakening: A Daily Guide to Conscious Living. By Shakti Gawain. A daily meditation guide that focuses on maintaining your spiritual center not just when you are in solitude, but when you are in the world, and especially, in relationships. (Trade paperback $8.95)

Embracing Our Selves: The Voice Dialogue Manual. By Drs. Hal and Sidra Stone. The highly acclaimed, groundbreaking work that explains the psychology of the selves and the Voice Dialogue method. (Trade paperback $12.95)

Embracing Each Other: Relationship as Teacher, Healer and Guide. By Drs. Hal and Sidra Stone. A compassionate guide to understanding and improving our relationships. The follow-up to the Stone's pioneering book on Voice Dialogue. (Trade paperback $11.95)

Maps to Ecstasy: Teachings of an Urban Shaman. By Gabrielle Roth with John Loudon. A modern shaman shows us how to reconnect to the vital energetic core of our being through dance, song, theater, writing, meditation, and ritual. (Trade paperback $9.95)

Notes from My Inner Child: I'm Always Here. By Tanha Luvaas. This deeply touching book puts us in contact with the tremendous energy and creativity of the inner child. (Trade paperback $8.95)

Coming Home: The Return to True Self. By Martia Nelson. A down-to-earth spiritual primer that explains how we can use the very flaws of our humanness to carry the vibrant energy of our true self and reach the potential that dwells in all of us. (Trade paperback $12.95)

Corporate Renaissance: Business as an Adventure in Human Development. By Rolf Osterberg. This groundbreaking book explodes the myth that a business's greatest asset is capital, and shows why employees must come first for businesses to succeed in the 90s. (Hardcover $18.95)

Passion to Heal: The Ultimate Guide to Your Healing Journey. By Echo Bodine. An invaluable guide for mapping out our individual journeys to health. (Trade paperback $14.95)

The Path of Transformation: How Healing Ourselves Can Change the World. By Shakti Gawain. Shakti gave us *Creative Visualization* in the 70s, *Living in the Light* in the 80s, and now *The Path of Transformation* for the 90s. Shakti's new bestseller delivers an inspiring and provocative message for the path of true transformation. (Trade paperback $9.95)

The Revelation: Our Crisis Is a Birth. By Barbara Marx Hubbard. An underground classic from one of the true prophets of our time. Hubbard offers an astounding interpretation of the Book of Revelation, which reveals the consciousness required by the human race, not only to survive, but to blossom into full realization of its potentials. (Trade paperback 365 pgs. $16.95)

Tapes

Living in the Light: Read by Shakti Gawain. Shakti reads her bestseller on developing intuition. (Two cassettes $15.95)

Developing Intuition. Shakti Gawain expands on the ideas about intuition she first discussed in *Living in the Light.* (One cassette $10.95)

The Path of Transformation: How Healing Ourselves Can Change the World. Shakti reads her inspiring new bestseller. (Two 70-minute cassettes $15.95)

To Place an Order

Call 1-800-949-1091.